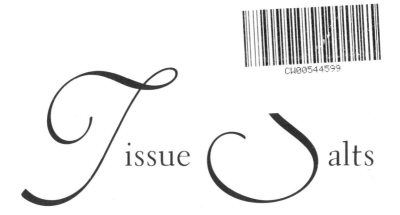

Tissue Salts

for Healthy Living

Margaret Roberts

Published by Struik Nature
(an imprint of Random House Struik (Pty) Ltd)
Reg. No. 1966/003153/07
Wembley Square, First Floor, Solan Road
Gardens, Cape Town 8001
PO Box 1144, Cape Town, 8000 South Africa

Visit us at **www.randomstruik.co.za** and subscribe
to our newsletter for monthly updates and news

First published in 2001 by Spearhead, an imprint of
New Africa Books (Pty) Ltd
This edition published in 2008 by Struik Nature

10 9 8 7 6

Managing editor: Reneé Ferreira
Copy-editor: Elsa Austin
Cover photographs: Phyllis Green
Cover design by Crazy Cat Designs
Design and typesetting by Alicia Arntzen, Lebone Publishing Services
Printed and bound by Pinetown Printers, Pinetown, KwaZulu-Natal.

ISBN 978 1 77007 773 7
Also available in Afrikaans as Weefselsoute vir Heilsaamheid 978 1 77007 774 4

Warning:
The content of this book is not intended as a substitute for consultation with
a medical professional. Do not undertake any course of treatment without
the advice of your doctor. The author and publishers take no responsibility
for any illness or discomfort that may result from information contained in
this book.

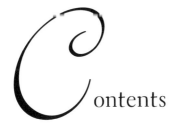

$\mathcal{C}$ontents

Acknowledgements iv

Introduction vi

What are tissue salts? viii

Tissue salts in a nutshell... x

The 12 Tissue Salts

  1. Calc. Fluor.: Calcium Fluoride.. 1

  2. Calc. Phos.: Calcium Phosphate... 8

  3. Calc. Sulph.: Calcium Sulphate 16

  4. Ferrum Phos.: Ferrum Phosphoricum................................... 24

  5. Kali. Mur.: Kaliu m Muriaticum... 32

  6. Kali. Phos.: Kalium Phosphate.. 40

  7. Kali. Sulph.: Kalium Sulphate 50

  8. Mag. Phos.: Magnesium Phosphate...................................... 57

  9. Nat. Mur.: Natrium Muriaticum 65

  10. Nat. Phos.: Natrium Phosphoricum 75

  11. Nat. Sulph.: Natrium Sulphate.. 83

  12. Silica: Silicon Dioxide 91

Ailment Chart 101

*A*cknowledgements

I have many people to thank for their help in my work with tissue salts. First and foremost my friend, Doreen Mankowitz, who introduced me to this wonderful way of self-help — she is a life changer, having shared her bounty of knowledge with so many of us over the years. To a loyal and supportive friend of long standing, my most grateful thanks.

To Natura Homeopathic Laboratories, in particular Dr. Elsabé Stoffberg and Mary Green, the manufacturers of the tissue salts I use, who warmly support us and respond to all our needs, with unstinting helpful advice and such kindness that make this sick old world a better place. Thank you for so much and for so professionally bottling all my last-minute orders. Your act is beautifully together.

For my publisher, Nicholas Combrinck, who lets me loose and free and gives me the rare chance to write a book — a life changer — such as this, my gratitude always.

To my editor, Reneé Ferreira, who drives kilometres to collect and dispatch manuscripts and who remains always the same — supportive and considerate. Thank you for not pressing and pushing the deadlines and for gathering it all together and keeping a cool head!

To my copy editor, Elsa Austin, editor of my years of magazine articles and who knows my writing so well. It has been pure pleasure to work with you, knowing you're as excited about the wonders of these salts as I am. Thank you for catching up the loose ends and for cross-indexing and keeping every fact in place!

To my three children and the farm animals and birds on whom I experimented and into whom I forced these 'little white pills' and dabbed on to them strange pale lotions. Thank you that you so obligingly opened little mouths and snouts and beaks, and for over 30 years gave me the extraordinary experience of astonishing results that ended up in this book! And look how healthy you all are and what well-balanced adults you've all grown into!

To Annatjie van Wyk, my clever-at-deciphering typist, who manages to cram into her busy schedule the results of my 4 a.m. scribblings, my midnight scrawlings and my rush and flurry and ASAP notes. She delivers on time every time, and keeps track of everything every day. Annatjie even remembers what I wrote last month! Thank you for saving me so often and for catching the fly-away pages I drop off at the farm gate in the dark dawns.

To Phyllis Green, the photographer, who gives so much time and shares so much interest in recording a picture library of every herb and plant mentioned in this book, and for taking the cover photographs. We all enjoy working with you!

I need also to mention the huge number of students who have attended my tissue salt classes at the Herbal Centre and whose lives have improved because of the salts and who have experienced and verified what I have written here. Thank you all for so enthusiastically giving me feedback.

I am filled with such gratitude that these natural, simple remedies can make such a difference in so many ways and in so many lives. It is all because of Dr. Schuessler's research and experiments so many decades ago, we can now benefit from nature and become whole and balanced and healthy throughout all the days of our lives.

Herbal Centre
De Wildt
North West Province
South Africa

Winter 2001

*I*ntroduction

This will probably be one of the most unusual books you will ever read and undoubtedly one of the most important books I will ever write.

My hope is that it will provide an enlightening and surprisingly simple, but new approach to health supplements. You may even find the outcome, after taking tissue salts, both astonishing and life-changing — even mind-blowing. For that is what the precious tissue salts can actually achieve. They will literally change your way of thinking about health, and how you will cope in future with every mood, every anxiety, from the day-to-day little ailments to the bigger, more frightening illnesses that relentlessly plague us and those near and dear to us.

The twenty-first century brings with it undreamt of problems and situations. Current conditions tax our bodies, our minds — our very souls — as we strive to keep pace with technology and the demands of life today. As a result, we are often in a state of such anxiety that it seems we'll never emerge to cope with future obstacles.

What we don't realise is that, due to intense stress, our bodies and minds have become depleted. But, by selecting the specific mineral salts our body needs, and correcting our diet to include the fruits, vegetables and herbs that are predominantly rich in these particular minerals, we can attain vibrant health, and an alert and positive mindset. And, best of all, we can cope with all that life has to offer while fighting illness and debilitation.

I first learnt about biochemic tissue salts well over 30 years ago when, expecting my second baby, I was suffering from morning sickness. I have my long-time special friend, Doreen Mankowitz, to thank for not only giving me so many inspiring books to read and for stimulating my mind so constantly, but also for introducing me to tissue salts through a book written by Dr. Carey and Dr. Perry, *The Salts of Salvation*. Doreen generously gave me all 12 of the tissue salts and watched while I took Kali. Mur., which immediately settled my morning sickness and Nat. Mur., which quickly cleared my hay fever. I have never looked back and, while I waded through the prolific 1932 edition of the publication (originally written in 1906), I developed a total fascination that has never left me.

According to the two doctor authors, there is no human condition that cannot be helped by the specific tissue salt for that ailment. And, through the years since then, I have proved this fact over and over again — not only for humans but also for animals, birds and even plants — with each incidence showing an immediate and often profound response. I wondered how I ever lived without them.

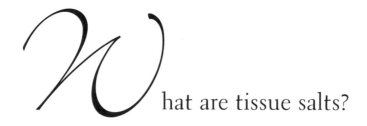

hat are tissue salts?

Tissue salts — also called cell salts or biochemic salts — are minerals, the same minerals that are found in the earth's rocks and soil. These minerals should be present in our bodies in a perfect balance, which is the prerequisite for complete health and well-being.

Dr. Schuessler (1828-1898), an eminent 19th century German physician, discovered upon analysis, that when the human cell is reduced to ashes, it exhibits 12 minerals. He named this system *biochemistry* (the chemistry of life) from the Greek word *bios* meaning 'the course of life' and *chemistry* which means the knowledge of the elements and the laws governing their combination and behaviour.

The tissue salts are present in our food, or should be, when grown organically in mineral-rich soils. But, in modern-day agricultural practices, soils are leached of their life-sustaining minerals and boosted instead with chemical fertilisers and fumigants.

Dr. Schuessler regarded the inorganic mineral substances that constitute our planet Earth as the complete basis of the composition of our body's bone and blood, organs and muscles. Ground down into minute particles, they could be easily absorbed by the human body.

Tissue salts can be bought from every pharmacy and health shop. Hand-ground in lactose over six attenuations, called 'trituration', the result is an easily absorbable pill that contains a minute amount of a specific mineral salt in a lactose base. For babies and diabetics, or for those who prefer a liquid form, six to 10 drops in a little water can be taken three to 10 times a day.

Recommended dosage

- As a general rule the tablet form is most commonly taken, two tablets two to four times a day.
- For acute conditions take two tablets crushed in a little warm water every 10 to 30 minutes to one hour. Once the condition eases, place two tablets under the tongue and let them dissolve, repeat every two to three hours during the day. Then every four to six hours until the condition clears.
- For chronic conditions take two tablets of a specific salt. Often there are two or three other salts needed for the condition, so take them a few minutes after each other, usually two at a time twice a day or even three times a day, held under the tongue to dissolve.

Are tissue salts safe? Can you overdose?

Perfectly safe, and no, you cannot overdose. Toxicity is just not possible — the concentration is microscopic, usually one part per million. For minor illnesses and ailments tissue salts are completely safe, but in any event **always consult your doctor before starting a home treatment.**

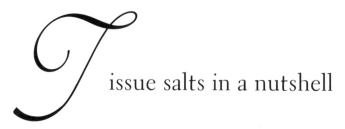

issue salts in a nutshell

Below is a concise synopsis of the main action or use of the 12 tissue salts — the key words associated with each salt here is the information usually offered on the bottle label.

 Calc. Fluor.: Elasticity; flexibility; toning; strength and resilience of muscular and connective tissue, bones, tooth-enamel and walls of the blood vessels.

 Calc. Phos.: A cell builder, this is an excellent tonic, and growth developer and supporter. It maintains body functions and aids recuperation. It is needed for blood, connective tissue, teeth and bones.

 Calc. Sulph.: Nature's cleanser and blood purifier, it dissolves discharge, drains tissues, heals and clears suppuration; an eliminator, it works particularly on the liver, blood, bile.

 Ferrum Phos.: The breath of life — the oxygen transporter; anti-inflammatory; anti-haemorrhage; cooler of inflamed, overheated conditions. It helps the formation of red blood corpuscles and strengthens the blood vessels. A first-aid remedy.

 Kali. Mur.: A superb tissue salt for children, specifically for childhood diseases; liver function; decongestant; anti-inflammatory; resolving the second stage of inflammation; glandular tonic; blood and lymphatic conditioner; a digestive. It is essential for the blood and nerve tissue.

Kali. Phos.: A nerve nutrient and natural tranquilliser, it lifts the spirits and restores a feeling of well-being; gives emotional balance; pain reliever; important for heart, brain tissue and intracellular fluid.

Kali. Sulph.: A cell oxygenator — with Ferrum Phos. it transports oxygen; supports liver function; works particularly well for skin conditions like eczemas, and the mucous membranes, which it normalises, clears and conditions; getting rid of mucous.

Mag. Phos.: The antispasmodic, natural pain reliever for cramps, a superb nerve and muscle relaxant and nutrient, it also treats spasms, tension, bladder stones and stress-related pains and tensions.

Nat. Mur.: For heavy emotions, anger, depression, irritability, this is also a water distributor salt for skin conditions, for runny nose, hay fever and all mucous membrane conditions.

Nat. Phos.: Nature's antacid and natural acid-alkaline balancer, it treats digestive complaints, arthritic pains and stiffness. Generally this is a mood lifter, system neutraliser and a stress reliever.

Nat. Sulph.: Nature's diuretic and toxin cleanser, it is a liver decongestant, and a regulator of body fluid in the whole metabolism.

Silica: It eliminates toxins from the tissues, clears suppuration, and expels foreign matter from the body. It also strengthens connective tissue, supports and sustains after excess stress and overwork, improves memory function and mineral assimilation — the perfect tissue salt for the not so young.

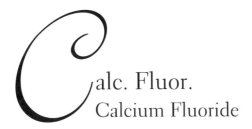

$\mathcal{C}$alc. Fluor.
Calcium Fluoride

$\mathcal{T}$his mineral salt is characterised by these words: elasticity, flexibility, toning mental faculties like indecisiveness. It proves excellent combined with other tissue salts, due to its toning ability, (i.e., toning of elastic fibres) which means it is of great importance in the treatment of skin ailments and circulatory problems. Calc. Fluor. is invaluable for both the growing child and the ageing adult.

Ailments treated

The skeleton
Take Calc. Fluor. for bone problems and the healing of fractures, for enlarged finger joints due to gout and rheumatism and for fatigue and pain in the lower back and a feeling of great weariness. For someone whose work depends on the strength of the back, putting it under constant strain, take two tablets of Calc. Fluor. alternating every four hours with two Nat. Mur. tablets. This is extremely helpful if taken daily for 14 days.

The teeth
If the mouth feels dry and there is much dental decay, this is the tissue salt to remember. For children with delayed dentition, Calc. Fluor. has been proven to be extremely beneficial. When the teeth feel loose in the sockets, don't delay, take Calc. Fluor. Dissolve four tablets in warm water or add 20 drops of the liquid form of the tissue salt to a glass of warm water. Use this to rinse the mouth out, holding it in the mouth and swishing around for as long as possible to achieve good contact with the gums. This will also help to ease

1

the sensitivity of the teeth to heat and cold and to build up deficient enamel. This is the most important salt for tooth enamel and to heal cracks in the tongue.

Slimming

Calc. Fluor. is an important slimming tissue salt, when two tablets are taken one hour before a meal, alternately with Calc. Phos. These two tissue salts will aid the assimilation of starches and fats and so minimise the build-up of fatty deposits.

The eyes

For cataracts, or hard cyst-like layers of cells on the eye surface, Calc. Fluor. will greatly help. This salt will quickly correct a delay in focusing when turning the head too quickly. For a nervous tick or pains in the eye, Calc. Fluor. is quickly soothing. When you've read for too long, straining the eyes when studying or the focus is blurred, take Calc. Fluor. every 15 minutes – just one tablet – for about an hour or so. For cataracts, alternate two tablets of Calc. Fluor. with two tablets of Calc. Phos. four times a day. Conjunctivitis responds quickly to Calc. Fluor., with Calc. Phos. and Nat. Mur., taken on the hour, one to two tablets of each – for about four to five hours. Spots before the eyes, flickering and light flashes can also be alleviated with Calc. Fluor. For ulcers and spots on the cornea, take two tablets of Calc. Phos. alternately with two tablets of Calc. Fluor. daily twice, or even three times. Calc. Fluor. also improves that feeling of pressure on the eyes.

Circulatory system, veins and haemorrhoids

Varicose veins and painful piles are two of Calc. Fluor.'s most marvellous areas of relief. The pain and throbbing is immediately eased and, for protruding piles, Calc. Fluor. helps to tone and shrink them. Soothe rectal fissures with a *cream* made by combining 10 Calc. Fluor. together with six Kali. Sulph. tablets, finely crushed and mixed into one cup of good aqueous cream. This ointment, applied frequently to the area, will give immediately relief. At the same time, take two of each tablet three times a day dissolved under the tongue. If piles are bleeding, take Ferrum Phos. as well. Six tablets Calc. Fluor. can also

2

be dissolved in ½ cup warm water and the solution applied to the area on cotton wool as a poultice and to soothe itching and irritation. Calc. Fluor. is also helpful in constipation where there is a chronic inability to expel faeces. It also helps to stop the bleeding of the lining of the anus and heals the little cracks around the stretched area.

The skin
Calc. Fluor. is excellent for chapped skin, fissures around the nails, the lips, the heels, in the palm of the hand and in eczemas where the skin weeps, hardens and cracks. Often when scars form and remain prominent, Calc. Fluor. can be taken with Silica. They can also be made into a *cream* – six tablets of each, crushed and finely mixed in ½ cup of aqueous cream. Add two teaspoons of vitamin E oil and one tablespoon almond oil and blend everything together well. This cream makes a superb massage balm if worked into the scar in small circular movements twice a day. It will soon break down scar tissue, dispersing and loosening it.

Digestive system
For those who suffer from hiccups, or with indigestion and the vomiting of undigested food, Calc. Fluor. will aid digestion and relieve spasms. Hold one tablet under the tongue after meals and let it dissolve. For children with hiccups, four to five drops of Calc. Fluor., in liquid form, on the tongue will quickly stop the spasms of hiccups.

Feminine problems
For menstrual flow that is too thick with large dark clots, Calc. Fluor. will resolve the problem. Sometimes, after a miscarriage, the uterus loses muscle tone and Calc. Fluor. tones and strengthens the tissues. This is one of its major functions, so taking two tablets of Calc. Fluor. twice daily is extremely important. When menstrual flow is excessive, with bouts of flooding, Calc. Fluor. can be taken four times a day, with immediate results. Often, with excessive menstruation, it is accompanied by a feeling that one's pelvic floor is falling out and sometimes there are bearing down pains. Alleviate both problems by lying on the back with knees bent and place a hot-

water bottle up against the pelvic floor. Take two Calc. Fluor. tablets under the tongue and rest for 15 minutes. Half an hour later take two more tablets and, if necessary, again after a further hour.

Respiratory system

For asthma sufferers Calc. Fluor. is wonderfully comforting, especially if there are signs of a productive cough. Take two tablets, placed under the tongue, every 15 minutes until the chest tightness goes. And, for a long-standing cold that just will not go away, accompanied by an irritating cough, post-nasal drip and a middle-ear infection – take two Silica tablets and twice or three times a day take two Calc. Fluor. tablets. It never fails to astonish me that such an easily administered, simple treatment can banish so much discomfort. This also works wonderfully for animals.

How you feel

So often ailments that really need Calc. Fluor. are associated with bad weather, especially during cold, damp conditions, chilly winds, draughts and damp, grey days. Some people are adversely affected by bad weather patterns. They show signs of depression, irritation and a host of other negative personality traits that exhibit a need for Calc. Fluor. A sad, restless, demotivated disposition can be greatly improved by taking two Calc. Fluor. tablets, held under the tongue until dissolved, and the symptoms will be relieved. Calc. Fluor. literally gives strength, steadiness, not only physically but mentally too. And, for schoolchildren who shows lack of concentration, instability, and erratic behaviour with tales of exaggerated fantasies, this is the 'coping' mineral so much needed in the frenetic world of today. People of all age groups endure stressful times but, by taking Calc. Fluor., many symptoms can be alleviated.

Growths and swellings

Cysts and bumps under the skin, fibroids in the uterus and odd growths under and on the skin, plus tissue overproduction, can often be dissolved by taking Calc. Fluor. on a regular and long-term basis. But, should any growth feel painful or a growth appear in the breasts, see your doctor without delay.

4

There have been several marvellous tales of Calc. Fluor. treating bone problems in horses. A magnificent pedigreed yearling had malformed, hugely ossified hoofs and knobbly joints in its forelegs. A team of veterinarians tried many treatments but without success, until one day an old doctor happened to see the horse. He prescribed Calc. Fluor. – 10 tablets twice a day for three months, then 10 tablets once a day for six months, and then six tablets every day for a year. The improvement was gradual but sustained and, within a year, the horse was sound, normal and had started being trained for polo. Today he is one of the great polo horses and is used for breeding.

The intestines
Hiatus hernia is a worrying and prevalent modern ailment, and distended bowel pockets in the colon often lead to irritable bowel syndrome – now a common problem. Constipation is a modern-day curse and a loss of tissue elasticity is diagnosed as the root cause for all these uncomfortable conditions that are inevitably due to a lack of Calc. Fluor. Two tablets three times a day will greatly improve the condition and tone the blood vessels.

Urinary system
Like the intestines, the bladder can be comfortingly soothed and the tissues toned and strengthened, particularly in the aged, by taking two tablets of Calc. Fluor. three times a day. This treatment is also recommended for an enlarged prostate gland and any tissue hardening in the area and around the urethra.

Sleep
Fearful, frightening nightmares and disturbing dreams can be put to rest by three tablets of Calc. Fluor., taken before you go to bed. Gentle stretching exercises will increase the circulation and help to unwind and relax body and mind.

Secondary and complementary salts
Silica works beautifully with Calc. Fluor. on all the above-mentioned symptoms, but particularly in bone disorders and overproduction of

tissue. Kali. Phos. is similar to Calc. Fluor. in its toning abilities and its mental brightening and mood-lifting quality. Include these two complementary salts – two tablets of each once a day, with Calc. Fluor.

Herbs that contain Calc. Fluor.

- Garlic: eat a clove a day either in food or in capsule form. Garlic is nature's antibiotic.
- Parsley: take one tablespoon fresh chopped parsley every day sprinkled on food. Parsley is a superb detoxifier, especially good for kidney and bladder ailments.
- Sage (*Salvia officinalis*): for brain power and to clear coughs, colds, sinus, 'flu, drink a cup of *sage tea* – ¼ cup fresh leaves in one cup of boiling water, stand five minutes, then strain, sweeten with a little honey if liked. Take one cup alternate days, or one cup daily or twice daily in acute conditions.
- Winter savory (*Satureja montana*): a wonderful digestive herb. Sprinkle ½ tablespoon fresh finely chopped leaves on meat and bean dishes. It will also ease muscular aches, help to clear sinuses and ease constipation.
- Chickweed (*Stellaria media*): a luscious self-seeding winter weed with tiny, succulent leaves. It is a superb treatment for rheumatism, gout, kidney and bladder ailments and a skin softener. Sprinkle ½ cup fresh leaves on salads and cheese dishes daily during its brief life cycle.
- Mustard: fresh leaves are a circulatory stimulant, excellent for bladder, bowels, catarrh and aching joints. Eat one cupful three times a week, adding to salads and stir-fries. The flowers are also edible, as are the green pods and the sprouts.
- Chives: nature's antibiotic – keeps the circulation going briskly and will boost the immune system. Eat ½ cup daily in salads.
- Buckwheat: high in precious rutin, which strengthens the walls of the blood vessels. Leaves and flowers are rich in minerals, especially Calc. Fluor., and it will tone the whole circulatory network and help to clear and open blocked sinuses, ears, and post-nasal drip. Eat a cupful of buckwheat greens daily until the infection clears.

- Lemon and lemon pith: squeeze lemon juice on everything and scrape out the pith – a teaspoon of pith daily will help nails and teeth and it is rich in bioflavonoids, which strengthen the walls of the blood vessels and help to clear catarrh and sinus blockages.

Foods rich in Calc. Fluor.

Grapes, oranges, pumpkin, squash, cabbage, onions, rye bread. Anyone with aching joints and gouty deposits and swollen joints should avoid wheat products and bread. Take rye bread instead. All the fruits and vegetables in this list are rich in beta-carotene, vitamins C, A, D and vitamin P to a small extent (in lemons, oranges and their pith). Their rich diversity of minerals and bioflavonoids act synergistically with Calc. Fluor., which means the body easily absorbs the Calc. Fluor. it requires to treat many ailments.

Interestingly, if most of these foods and herbs were not included in the diet, the greater majority of the symptoms listed would unmistakeably be evident. Grow all the herbs and foods organically to keep the body at maximum health. Include at least 60 to 80 per cent of the listed foods and herbs in the diet daily.

 The constitutional tissue salt

In accordance with the writings of Dr. Perry and Dr. Carey, Calc. Fluor. is the constitutional salt most needed by Cancerians. Two tablets daily dissolved under the tongue should keep the critical balance of good health in check, should there be none of the above symptoms evident. Through the years I have found that by taking your own constitutional salt, many small problems are kept at bay. I am a Cancerian and when I've forgotten to take Calc. Fluor. for a few days, I see a whole set of little symptoms building up, starting with a crack at the corners of my mouth. But once I again take Calc. Fluor. tablets regularly, everything normalises and symptoms quickly disappear. Pay attention to this, for through past years I've run many experiments on the constitutional salts and find their uses amazingly accurate.

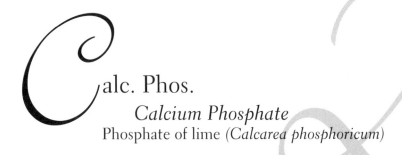

C alc. Phos.
Calcium Phosphate
Phosphate of lime *(Calcarea phosphoricum)*

This mineral salt is characterised by the following functions: cell builder and proliferator, growth supporter and developer, tonic, recuperation, restoration, builder of teeth, bones and nails.

Calc. Phos. intensifies the effect of other cell salts and it is one of the cell salts to take when you are feeling low, both in spirit and energy levels. It will help to give that necessary emotional lift, promoting healthy cellular activity while restoring tone to the whole system. The tonic effect of Calc. Phos. is so positive it has been named 'the body's chief building material'.

Ailments treated

The skeleton
During past years, when I worked as a physiotherapist, a Swiss doctor once taught me that Calc. Phos. is the most important tissue salt for aiding both physical and mental development in children. It is especially good for treating growing pains, rickets, for green stick fractures, shin soreness and for brittle bones and backache. He prescribed a tablet of Calc. Phos., to be sucked four times a day, for children who were slow developers. The same treatment was recommended for treating babies whose fontanelles (gaps in babies' sculls) were slow in closing, and also for those who showed signs of poor memory, bad temper and slow mental development. Calc. Phos. was given to children who slept badly, and whose limbs twitched at night. It also worked for others who woke, crying about sore shins and joints, or who had severe cramps and slow dentition. His patients' symptoms eased remarkably.

8

Slow-healing fractures, aches due to rheumatism and numbness in the bones, and stiffness due to coldness or poor circulation all respond well to Calc. Phos.. And, ageing animals with stiff, aching joints are also helped, particularly by a twice-daily dose of four to six tablets of Calc. Phos. A natural form of calcium that is easily absorbed, Calc. Phos. is essential for all degrees of osteoporosis – I am surprised that most doctors overlook this remarkable mineral. It is easily assimilated and properly utilised by all age groups, including the fast-ageing group of over 50-year-olds. It is important to understand that Calc. Phos. has a chain reaction effect on the bones with the ability to assimilate and fully absorb calcium in foods and especially in milk products.

The teeth
With adequate amounts of Calc. Phos. taken, dental caries is controlled remarkably well. Normal dental development and structural development of the mouth, delayed dentition and impacted teeth all respond quickly to a two or three times a day dose of Calc. Phos. For teething pains and fretfulness in babies, frequently use the liquid form of this salt, rubbing the drops gently on to the gums. Combined with Calc. Fluor. for inflamed, pale or bleeding gums, or for rapid tooth decay, Calc. Phos. is vitally important. One to two tablets of both Calc. Fluor. and Calc. Phos. twice or three times a day is the general dose.

Slimming
Calc. Phos. with Calc. Fluor. are the two tissue salts that, in combination, will help those wishing to rid their bodies of excess fat by helping to quell a ravenous appetite. Take two tablets of each, an hour before a meal – take them alternately – and they will assist in assimilation of the food while helping to disperse fatty deposits. But do follow a sensible eating plan – no tissue salts can keep you slim if you eat incorrectly.

The eyes
This is a most helpful cell salt when over-sensitivity to light is experienced, and also for eye twitches, pink eye (conjunctivitis) and

for flashing lights at the periphery of the eye. Many homeopathic doctors see a positive role for Calc. Phos. in the prevention and slowing of the progress of cataracts. For aching and stiffness behind the eyeballs – all the better for closing the eyes and putting gentle pressure on them – Calc. Phos. is indicated. If, when reading, there is visual distortion, take two tablets of Calc. Phos. four times a day. Similarly, if a cold feeling at the back of the eyes is experienced, or there are ulcers and spots on the cornea, the same dosage of Calc. Phos. will help to alleviate the symptoms.

Circulatory system

Chilblains, numb, cold hands and feet, cramps in cold limbs and chilliness – all these typical winter ills can be greatly alleviated by taking Calc. Phos. For clammy hands and the feeling of pins and needles, take two tablets of Calc. Phos. four times a day. If limbs feel as if they are asleep, take two tablets of Calc. Phos., followed in 20 minutes by another two. Repeat the dose two hours later – sucking the tablets slowly – to relieve these symptoms. Calc. Phos. and Nat. Mur., taken together, will help to restore normal energy to those suffering from low blood pressure. Two tablets of each, twice or three times a day is the recommended dose.

Digestive system

I have found Calc. Phos. extremely helpful for children with a poor appetite. Remember the cell salts can also be administered in liquid form, which is ideal for little children and for babies with colic. Four to six drops in a teaspoon of water does the trick and can be given every 10-15 minutes until symptoms subside.

Combined with Nat. Phos. and Mag. Phos., Calc. Phos. is excellent to ease burning indigestion, bloating and flatulence. I keep Calc. Phos. and Mag. Phos. near at hand for any spasmodic digestive disturbance and take two tablets of each as I go to bed if I've had a late dinner, eaten out, or had spicy or rich food. For acidity I combine these two with Nat. Phos. and it works like a charm.

Calc. Phos. eases irritable bowel syndrome when taken with Kali. Phos. and Nat. Sulph. And, to quell that constant craving for salty and savoury foods, combine it with Nat. Mur.

Feminine problems

When Calc. Phos. is lacking in the system, menstrual cramps often come to the fore, especially in teenagers or girls who are growing fast. Combined with Mag. Phos., one tablet of each taken frequently until the cramps subside is comforting. I found that by taking both, four times a day for two days prior to my period, I could alleviate a lot of pain and discomfort.

During pregnancy, Calc. Phos. is essential to the development of healthy bones in babies. It should be taken in conjunction with Mag. Phos., which helps to alleviate the mother's discomfort and cramp. During this time calcium is in huge demand and, unless it is replenished, this important mineral will be drained from the mother's bones, causing the start of osteoporosis in later life. Take two tablets of Calc. Phos., twice or three times a day during and after pregnancy, while feeding the baby.

Calc. Phos. helps women to carry a baby to full term. It is also recommended for women who have had trouble falling pregnant due to suppressed or irregular menstruation – often associated with anaemia or a faulty diet. And, for girls who are too young to be menstruating and women who are going into menopause, Calc. Phos. is a wonderful regulator. Dr. Schuessler found Calc. Phos. to be a particularly helpful women's cell salt and advised that all women should take it twice daily during menstruation.

Calc. Phos. and the Pill

Calc. Phos. is also an antidote for side-effects of the Pill. This method of birth control has been a bone of contention for many women who have experienced weight gain or weight loss, malfunctioning thyroid and changes in their breasts, not to mention the seesaw of emotions felt. Calc. Phos. is extremely helpful for women who have stopped taking the Pill, as it will once again help to restore normal menstruation.

Respiratory system

For those of us who catch cold easily, or are prone to recurrent and chronic bronchitis, pneumonia, tonsillitis, chronic cough and nasal catarrh, Calc. Phos. is indicated. In the case of enlarged adenoids or tonsils, and constant post-nasal drip allied to frequent ear, nose and throat infections – particularly in children – and chronic phlegm with albuminous nose mucous, one tablet taken three or four times a day quickly brings relief.

If children suffer from a rough, hoarse voice and nasal polpi, if the tongue feels stiff and numb and if there is a bad taste in the mouth in the mornings with foetid breath, the need for Calc. Phos. is indicated. It will also ease a sore, swollen throat when it is too painful to swallow and breathing feels tight and uncomfortable. Crush and dissolve six tablets of Calc. Phos. in ½ glass of warm water, or add 20 drops of liquid Calc. Phos. to the water. Frequently sip a little very slowly, letting it trickle down the throat.

Urinary system

Taking Calc. Phos. can quickly solve problems of bed-wetting, restless sleep and nightmares in children. Combine it with Kali. Phos. and Mag. Phos. if there are also growing pains and sore joints. Bladder and kidney stones, composed of calcium compounds, respond well to Calc. Phos. as it helps to break down acidity. When combined with Nat. Phos. and taken frequently, there is usually relief.

Mental problems

Calc. Phos. is recommended in cases of poor concentration, for moody anger and aggressiveness, when children are fretful, peevish or whining. It is also effective when there seems to be a severe incapacity of coherent thought and for problems at school when youngsters fail to concentrate or follow the teacher. This cell salt, taken three times a day, will greatly assist the development of a better mental state – for all age groups. And, when taken in conjunction with Mag. Phos. (which is closely related to Calc. Phos.) the child should be happier, quieter and more tolerant.

Apart from a noticeable improvement in the disposition of children, Calc. Phos. also works wonders for the aged, particularly in the disturbing times of change, grief and adjustment to loss, and it improves the memory. It works well for elderly folk who have become depressed and fearful at their advancing ageing, general helplessness and occurrence of heart palpitations. Calc. Phos. with Kali. Phos. are the two cell salts that combine to lift the mood and sense of wellbeing. Taken regularly, Calc. Phos. helps people to cope, diminishing that feeling of dread and internal tension.

The head

Headaches with coldness the sharp stabbing pain in the head that comes when directly exposed to cold air, aching sinuses, children's headaches, puberty and pregnancy headaches, and ear ache that occurs following exposure to the cold all warn that Calc. Phos. is depleted. Two tablets under the tongue every 10-15 minutes will swiftly ease the pain and the feelings of cold.

The skin

When there's a calcium deficiency, the complexion looks pasty, pimply and unhealthy. Calcium is needed to make the skin glow, and if the scalp also shows signs of hair loss and flaking, there is a deficiency in Calc. Phos.. Teenage acne, rough red spots and swollen lymph glands in the neck all respond to long-term treatment, namely a tablet of Calc. Phos., taken three times a day.

Secondary and complementary salts

Mag. Phos. and Calc. Phos. are superb antispasmodics and structural cell salts and, when taken in conjunction with Silica, the body becomes structurally stronger. Calc. Phos. is often referred to as the 'raw building material' and Silica as nature's refining 'sculptor', distributing calcium smoothly around the body.

Kali. Mur., when taken with Calc. Phos., is excellent in aiding recovery from bronchitis and pneumonia. And, with Ferrum Phos. and Calc. Phos. together, anaemia is greatly improved. These two salts are superb for circulatory weakness and chilliness.

Herbs that contain Calc. Phos.

In all my years of working with tissue salts, I never fail to be astonished at how correctly the herbs that contain the necessary components do exactly what the corresponding tissue salt does! For instance:

13

- Comfrey has the ability to build bones (it is commonly called 'knit-bone'), and it also clears chest ailments such as pneumonia and bronchitis. It also helps to strengthen the back (the skeleton in general), it clears kidney infections and is anti-ageing. Note: Comfrey is now considered unsafe to take internally and this old-fashioned herb is now banned in some countries. Consult your doctor before taking comfrey.
- Chamomile is a sedative, calming, unwinding and de-stressing herb that helps to clear kidney and digestive ailments while strengthening sluggish circulation and soothing aches and pains. A cup of *chamomile tea* will soothe the anxieties of the day beautifully and is rich in calcium! Add ¼ cup fresh sprigs of flowers to one cup of boiling water. Allow to stand for five minutes, strain, sweeten with honey and sip just before bedtime. Or, add two teaspoons of dried flowers to one cup of boiling water, stir until it starts to colour – about four to five minutes.
- Lucerne (alfalfa) used fresh in salads, both leaves and flowers, or as a tea (made as above), is another strengthening energiser. Rich in calcium, it boosts the circulation and clears infection, pain and strains while boosting the immune system.
- Borage leaves, flowers and seeds are all rich in calcium and can be added to soups and stews, or made into teas (as above). It is particularly helpful when used to treat coughs, feverish stages of pneumonia, bronchitis and 'flu. Mixed with a little honey and lemon juice, borage makes an excellent cough and throat treatment.
- Oats – the traditional breakfast food of Europe – is rich in calcium and is a restorative, bone building, nerve tonic that also helps to reduce blood cholesterol. Oatstraw, the ripened dried stems and leaves and ripe grain, can also be made into a *tea*. Use ¼ cup dried chopped straw and a few oats seeds. Pour over one cup of boiling water. Stand five minutes, strain, sweeten with a little honey if liked. Take one to two cups daily as an anti-depressant, restorative tonic, for building bone and to relieve osteoporosis.

All the above-mentioned herbs are easy to grow – it is really worthwhile having your own herb garden close at hand.

14

Foods rich in Cal. Phos.

Include in the daily diet at least eight items from this important list:

- Green leafy vegetables – lettuces, spinach and cabbage particularly.
- Carrots, lentils, strawberries, mulberries, raspberries, cranberries, figs, plums.
- All the whole grains you enjoy – oats porridge, barley water, wheat sprouts, alfalfa sprouts.
- Dairy products, particularly plain Bulgarian yoghurt and cottage cheese, and at least a glass of milk daily.
- Lean meat grilled (not fried), or stewed, is also rich in calcium, and so are eggs.

 The constitutional tissue salt

Calc. Phos. is the tissue salt most needed by people born under the astrological sign of Capricorn. Capricorns need to build a positive attitude and this essential cell salt is the building material of the body, and a superb stabiliser of the nervous system. I never cease to be amazed at how each constitutional salt fits so exactly and so perfectly with the personality born under a specific astrological time period. As Dr. Carey and Dr. Perry so cleverly pointed out, never was there a cell salt more essential to the restructuring and restoring of individual lives so that each one of us – and particularly those born under the astrological sign of Capricorn – feels safer, supported and nurtured. The feel-good-all-over quality imparted by Calc. Phos. is vitally important for those under this sign of the zodiac.

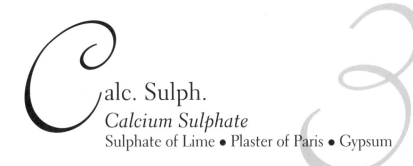

Calc. Sulph.
Calcium Sulphate
Sulphate of Lime • Plaster of Paris • Gypsum

Calc. Sulph. is characterised by the following functions: Blood cleanser and purifier, suppuration reducer and eliminator. It is found in the blood, the body's connective tissue, the bile, the liver and in the epithelial cells in the skin.

A rejuvenating cell salt, it literally cleans out the body, destroying old cells, abnormal discharges (pus, mucous and chronic infections) while hastening the healing and cleansing of wounds, catarrh, inflammations and ulcers.

This is the mineral used to make plaster casts – it is commonly known as Plaster of Paris. It is naturally present in eggshells and is used by farmers as lime sulphate to build up the soil. It gives colour to grapes and, in the last century, was an essential soil constituent in every vineyard across the world.

Dr. Carey and Dr. Perry found that when combined with Silica – which is known as the biochemical surgeon – Calc. Sulph. should follow after Silica, as the latter cell salt promotes pus formation in the healing process. Calc. Sulph. clears pus, and will actually stop a wound from discharging pus if used early enough! The two doctors found the combination of Silica and Calc. Sulph. quite remarkable in its cleansing action.

Ailments treated

The skin
In my early study of biochemic tissue salts, I kept coming across the words 'consider Calc. Sulph. first when there is an eruption of any

kind'. I have always followed this teaching, applying it to everything from acne to fever blisters, from a persistent deep-seated discharge that refuses to heal, to skin suppuration. Even a slow healing wound, boil or abscess, all will benefit from a three or even six-times-a-day dose of Calc. Sulph. (two tablets dissolved under the tongue). At the same time, apply a *topical application* comprising 10 tablets crushed and mixed with ½ cup of warm water. Dab the solution on to the area, spray it on from a spritz-action bottle or use it as a wash. Alternatively, 20 drops of Calc. Sulph. (in liquid form) added to ½ cup warm water can be applied directly.

It is also used for eczema, rashes, herpes and genital herpes, pimples that come to a head, adult late-onset acne and discharging crusts on the scalp. It clears dandruff, pimples that form a rash, as a result of shaving and a raw sore beard – especially in teenage boys just starting to shave. It treats boils, cuts and, most important, slow healing ulcers and suppurating insect bites, scratches, and similar wounds. All these symptoms indicate the body's need for Calc. Sulph., and all will benefit by external application of the solution in addition to taking the tablets orally. Remember, Calc. Sulph. is the key tissue salt in the prevention of new infection.

The eyes
As a physiotherapist, I was exposed to a varied range of unusual ailments. Research doctors had found that improving the circulation to the face, neck and chest assisted the healing of several severe cases of pustular acne. One doctor used a paste of oatmeal with Calc. Sulph. that proved excellent for cleansing the area. Similarly, two of the patients' pink eye (conjunctivitis) symptoms cleared up at the same time.

Only many years later did I discover that Calc. Sulph. clears eye infections and the subsequent yellow discharges in the corners of the eyes as well as deep ulcers, abrasions and scratches on the cornea of the eyes. It also clears watery eyes and continual tears. Two tablets taken three to six times a day during the inflammatory stage will ease the condition considerably, and twice a day thereafter, until all symptoms have disappeared.

17

The ears

Calc. Sulph. should be taken for catarrh and blocked, ringing ears and continual wax production – especially dark wax – and in cases of persistent earache. A tablet should be taken up to six times a day. At the same time, a crushed tablet (dissolved in warm water as described above) should be applied with a swab of cotton wool to clean the ears and wash around the outer ear.

The mouth

For bleeding gums, gum boils and painful mouth ulcers, 20 drops of liquid Calc. Sulph. in half a cup of warm water, used frequently as a mouth wash, will quickly soothe the condition, and two tablets sucked four to six times a day will do much to clear all mouth ailments.

The respiratory tract

Take Calc. Sulph. in conjunction with Kali. Sulph. for persistent and recurring sore throat, tonsillitis, a continual discharge from the nose and a recurrent cough with sputum. It also treats a coated tongue, a blocked nose and sinuses, and the last stages of bronchitis where thick yellow sputum is evident. In cases of pneumonia, where there is endless coughing, swelling and tightness of the throat and a pressing pain when swallowing, Calc. Sulph. is sure to ease the symptoms when taken as described above.

Note: For serious respiratory ailments, Calc. Sulph. and Silica alone are often not enough – take the medicines prescribed by your doctor as well. The cell salts will help to clear up infection and hasten the healing. Calc. Sulph. has the ability to prevent a sore throat and the onset of a threatening cold, if taken frequently, together with Ferrum Phos., at the very first symptoms.

Digestive system

At one time or another, we have all experienced a craving for a particular type of food. Those who have a persistent craving for salty, savoury or sour foods need to take Calc. Sulph. Have you ever heard of the 'Coke and chips' syndrome? The saltiness of the chips, washed down with iced cola, is a pretty common craving. But

18

when it's five or six times a day, this is a signal that there is a real lack of Calc. Sulph. Two tablets taken three or four times a day will stop that intense craving. It is also useful for stomach ulcers, burning indigestion, a sudden ravenous appetite and, strangely enough, Calc. Sulph. is also indicated for people with no appetite at all. Even symptoms such as an aversion to coffee, milk or meat, or a desire for any sweet liquids due to a sudden terrible thirst are quickly eased by a couple of Calc. Sulph. tablets placed under the tongue, gently sucked, and the dose repeated three, four (or even five) times a day.

Calc. Sulph.: constipation and diarrhoea

Another use for Calc. Sulph. is in treating constipation and diarrhoea, particularly in chronic conditions. So often with these complaints a painful anal fistula forms that is slow to heal. Calc. Sulph., applied as a lotion as well as taken in tablet form, has proved effective. For children with diarrhoea, when the stool is dry and straw-coloured, Calc. Sulph. taken every half hour – one tablet at a time until the diarrhoea stops – will quickly ease the condition. But, be sure to consult a doctor if the condition persists and take Calc. Sulph. in conjunction with the prescribed medicine.

Sleeplessness

Insomnia is a worldwide problem. I am continually asked how to relieve the inability to sleep naturally and, along with the phosphates numbered '2', '4', '6', '8' and '10', I find Calc. Sulph. very helpful. Many people suffer at night from restlessness. The desire for sleep may come early, but then you awake around midnight, when all the depressing thoughts, the anxieties of the day, the heavy heart and the frightening anxious dreams engulf you. Get up and make yourself a cup of warm milk with a touch of honey. Fill a hot-water bottle – especially if your feet are chilled and you feel cold, shaky and scared. Then dissolve two tablets of Calc. Phos., two of Calc. Sulph. and two of Kali. Phos. in the warm milk, take the drink back to bed and sip it slowly.

If the bloodstream is full of old, toxic cells the body is trying to get rid of, allied to a deficiency of Calc. Sulph., these old, worn-out cells accumulate from long-standing infections. As a result, the general state of health is one of general 'unwellness' that can reflect in moodiness, an almost chronic anxiety, groundless fears, irritability and an overactive, cluttered and confused mind.

Even frontal headaches and nausea can waken you. The mind is correspondingly toxic and, for older people, this becomes a chronic worry. Always remember that this tissue salt helps to resolve and clear worn-out toxic conditions. Once we understand the slow healing process, and we know that cold, damp weather makes it worse, or an over-warm room also exacerbates it, we can set about coping with it. Taking Calc. Sulph., with a diet of fresh fruits, vegetables plus lots of gentle exercise and fresh air, will greatly ease and clear the condition.

Circulatory system

The liver is where worn-out cells and 'dis-eased' cells are cleared – a detoxification process. Without Calc. Sulph., the effectiveness of the elimination of the old cells is delayed. The waste products, having completed their life cycle, now end up in the liver and with insufficient Calc. Sulph. present, the liver becomes clogged and sluggish and skin eruptions result. If the deficiency of Calc. Sulph. extends into the connective tissues, those same eruptions are most likely to become an ulcer, a slow healing boil, an abscess or even a carbuncle. Varicose ulcers that become chronic can be alleviated by using a lotion of Calc. Sulph. and taking two tablets four times a day. This is very useful for the elderly person whose feet feel cold, and for varicosities that throb and are even ulcerated. Combined with Silica, Calc. Sulph. can work wonders.

A burning sensation under the feet combined with aching limbs has plagued so many people but, by taking a few tablets – usually 12 – over a period of two to three days, sufferers are always surprised at the relief Calc. Sulph. brings to ease this complaint.

Pancreas, liver and kidneys

In the roles of cleansing and detoxifying the body, Calc. Sulph. is of vital importance. As children, when we became quarrelsome or irritable and headachy, my grandmother called it 'being liverish'. Only many years later did I understand that these symptoms occur when Calc. Sulph. is depleted. Conditions such as bladder ailments, kidney soreness, muscular aches and pains and double vision can all become so prominent that we frequently urgently seek professional help when, in fact, they can be corrected by taking Calc. Sulph. three or four times a day for several days.

Homeopathic doctors suggest taking Calc. Sulph. as well as Mag. Phos. to counteract the bad side-effects of taking coal-tar medication like aspirin and other painkillers. Too many of these medications puts more strain on the liver, which gradually destroys the natural chemistry of the blood, thus leaving the body open to infections. So consider Calc. Sulph. an important detoxifier for the liver, kidneys and pancreas.

Secondary and complementary salts

The main one here is Silica with Calc. Sulph. – both work together for recurring, as well as chronic discharge anywhere in the body. Kali. Sulph. is very similar in action to Calc. Sulph., so study the symptoms and address both the detoxifying and cleansing of the body in addition to the emotional cleansing – these three tissue salts in combination often work like a charm.

Herbs that contain Calc. Sulph.

- Stinging nettle (*Uritica dioica*) is one of the most important herbs, and is rich in Calc. Sulph. The main action of nettle is cleansing and detoxifying. It is an excellent diuretic and increases urine production. It helps heal skin conditions, such as bites and infected sores, aids poor kidney function and alleviates fluid retention. Nettle is anti-allergenic, flushing toxins and waste from the liver. For arthritic conditions and gout, together with nasal problems (like rhinitis and hay fever), nettle remains one of the best healing herb treatments, having an excellent tonic action on the blood. To make *nettle tea* use ¼ cup fresh leaves in one cup boiling

21

water. Stand five minutes and then strain. Take one or two cups daily until the condition clears. Note: Wear gloves when handling the nettle plant.

- Red clover (*Trifolium pratense*): rich in minerals, especially calcium compounds and silica, red clover is an anti-spasmodic, a diuretic, an anti-inflammatory and it can be made into a syrup to clear phlegmy coughs. It also makes an excellent eye wash for treating conjunctivitis. Use it also in a douche for vaginal infections and to curb itching experienced during menopause. Use the flowers, crushed, to soothe and clear inflamed insect stings and rashes. A compress of leaves and flowers eases arthritic and kidney pains. To make a *tea*: add ¼ cup of fresh leaves and flowers to one cup of boiling water. Stand for five minutes, then strain and drink (one to two cups a day only). Use the same recipe as a *douche* or *lotion*.

- Wormwood (*Artemesia absinthium*): wormwood must be taken only under professional supervision. It is an old, much revered herb used for eliminating worms, for easing stomach pain and to stimulate the secretion of bile. Because it has an anti-inflammatory action, it helps to clear swelling and infections.

Foods rich in Calc. Sulph.

Every one of the following foods helps to fight infections:

- Onions, garlic, leeks are high in Calc. Sulph. – all boost the immune system and fight infection, help to clear persistent coughs and wounds that won't heal while helping to rid the body of toxins.

- Radishes, watercress, asparagus, cauliflower all assist in ridding the body of toxins while boosting circulation and each acts as a cleanser, toner and tonic.

- Figs and prunes are rich in calcium and specially help to eliminate waste.

- Also include celery, parsley and fennel. Take them in teas and in soups and salads daily, and the healing ability of the body will improve naturally and dramatically.

- Green salads and barley water are two health cleansers that should become part of your daily health ritual. To make *barley water*: gently boil one cup of pearl barley in two litres of water for about 40 minutes. Top up with water if necessary. Stand aside and cool. Strain and store in the refrigerator. Eat the grains like rice with lemon juice and drink two glasses of barley water daily with a dash of fresh fruit juice to give it flavour.

 The constitutional tissue salt

This is the tissue salt most needed by people born under the astrological sign of Scorpio. Typically, those born under the sign of Scorpio are more prone to toxaemia than other signs and, for this reason, Calc. Sulph. is particularly important as part of their daily health regime. Dr. Schuessler advised, over a hundred years ago, that heavy, worried, 'toxic' emotions could cause blockages and slow healing within the body. He suggested Calc. Sulph. as an effective eliminator.

Calc. Sulph. is a blood purifier, it clears waste and dissolves and eliminates discharge of every kind and Scorpios often suffer from ailments that can benefit from this sort of action. A diet rich in the above foods and herbs, and this exceptional cleansing and purifying tissue salt, will assist in promoting that state of well-being for which we all strive.

23

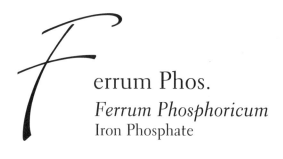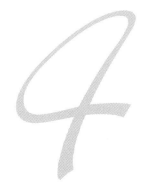

errum Phos.
Ferrum Phosphoricum
Iron Phosphate

Iron is contained in the haemoglobin of the blood and, to a great extent, in all the cells of the body except the actual nerves. But, the nerves are lined with a protective sheath – a connective tissue containing blood, which with its iron content is able to actually penetrate the cells to nourish them.

The haemoglobin of the blood is made up of protein, globulin and iron, and this is the combination that is able to process the oxygen in the blood and allow the carbon dioxide in the tissues to be released and returned to the lungs. Interestingly, iron with Kali. Sulph. carries life-giving oxygen all around the body to every cell, every tissue. Even more interesting is that it is the very presence of iron in the tissues, that activates all sorts of processes within the body, specially the all-important one of releasing energy from the food we eat.

Whenever there is even the slightest sign of infection or inflammation, Ferrum Phos. is the most important tissue salt to take. The key functions of Ferrum Phos. are anti-infection and anti-inflammatory and it can dramatically ease inflamed conditions. It is literally the primary first-aid remedy.

Ferrum Phos. is able to strengthen the walls of the bloodvessels, specially the main arteries – the body's freeways – and their ability to distribute fresh, oxygen-rich blood to the cells.

One point that needs to be stressed and remembered is that Ferrum Phos. is not solely a cure for anaemia. Anaemia is a complicated ailment that must be treated by a doctor, and iron may be needed as a supplement in homeopathic or in biochemic tissue salt form. Iron is vitally important and it works in subtle ways and, in the long run, these tiny frequent doses build up and lead to a profound effect. But, it is still extremely important to consult your doctor. If you are deficient in iron, the picture is one of a pale, lack-lustre, anaemic looking child, or a pale lack-lustre florid faced adult with no get-up-and-go energy or initiative, allied to a general listlessness, depression and mood of dejection.

Ailments treated

The head

When there are attacks of dizziness, fainting, fever, a flushed face, nose bleeds, throbbing headaches, high temperature, a ruddy complexion, a feeling of congestion, congestive headaches and a susceptibility to over-exertion of the brain, Ferrum Phos. will bring instant relief. Dissolve two tablets slowly under the tongue and take two more half an hour later, until the symptoms ease.

Infections

Ferrum Phos. is specifically recommended at the first stage of any illness or disease or injury – two tablets taken every 15 to 30 minutes for a couple of hours and then every hour until the symptoms subside. For children and, by the way, for animals too, one tablet taken as above is effective. Remember, iron carries oxygen that assists healing.

The eyes

Bloodshot, inflamed eyes, with a burning sensation, or a gritty feeling, as if sand was scraping over the eyeball at every blink, is frequently a sign that conjunctivitis is setting in and one to two tablets of Ferrum Phos., taken every 20-30 minutes, will ease the symptoms.

The ears

For earache and inflamed throbbing – if the outer ear is red and if a child complains of sore ears – Ferrum Phos. will help to resolve the condition effectively. A tablet, dissolved under the tongue, should be taken every 20 minutes, but do consult your doctor if the pain persists.

The teeth and gums

Any inflamed, swollen area in the mouth, ulcers on the gums or on the tongue, will quickly respond to Ferrum Phos. If baby is teething, rub the gums with liquid Ferrum Phos., Mag. Phos. and Calc. Phos. Add 10 drops of each to a little water, stir well then give a teaspoon of this mixture for baby to swallow. For toothache, take Ferrum Phos. and Mag. Phos. – two tablets of each – frequently until you can get to a dentist. Also, after a tooth extraction, make a mixture of two teaspoonfuls of salt and six crushed dissolved Ferrum Phos. tablets with six dissolved Mag. Phos. tablets mixed into a cup of warm water. Gently swish the mouth out with this soothing mixture every hour and it will quickly repair the hole left by the removed tooth.

Respiratory system

At the first sign of a sore throat, or shortness of breath associated with colds, bronchitis and tonsillitis, and the initial clear streaming nose as a cold begins, take Ferrum Phos. with Calc. Sulph. and Kali. Sulph. (one tablet of each) every 20 minutes for about three hours and then every hour following until the symptoms subside. The same remedy applies to those people suffering with chronic nasal and chest infections involving mucous and coughs.

Pregnancy

If you experience nausea and vomit easily, two tablets of Ferrum Phos. with Kali. Mur. taken four times a day will ease morning sickness. One tablet each of Nat. Phos., Nat. Sulph. and Ferrum Phos. will ease the incontinence (that involuntary urine spurt and general inability to hold the urge to urinate during pregnancy) most expectant mothers seem prone to suffer from.

The heart and circulatory system

If there is palpitation or rapid pulse, painful beating of the heart, a rush of blood to the head, flushed face, fever and associated overheating, a tendency to bleeding (nose bleeds especially), and for haemophilia patients, Ferrum Phos. is essential. When there is excessive bleeding with an injury or, if there is poor circulation, with cold hands and feet, or sign of blood in either diarrhoea or firm stools, Ferrum Phos. is vital. Two tablets taken every 15 minutes until the symptoms subside, is the usual dose. Take one to two tablets thereafter, three to four times a day.

Digestive system

Ferrum Phos. is one of the best digestive remedies, especially for nausea, diarrhoea and undigested stools. This was the one remedy I found helpful in treating multiple food allergies (intolerance) in children, especially when vomiting undigested milk, or sour belching and projectile vomiting. For a baby, a mixture of 10 drops in a little water quickly soothes constipation and all the above ailments.

Female problems

For irregular (or every three weeks) menstruation, with excessive bleeding, Ferrum Phos. is a great help. But, it must be taken regularly throughout the month, usually two tablets three times a day (combined with Mag. Phos. for cramps). To treat haemorrhoids (also for men), especially when they bleed, wash the area with a solution of 20 drops Ferrum Phos. in a little warm water, and take two tablets orally four times a day.

Menopause

To alleviate the symptoms of hot flushes, swollen feet or hands, water retention, night sweats, vertigo, and a florid complexion, two tablets of Ferrum Phos. should be taken four to eight times a day. If there is a sudden increase in blood pressure, take Ferrum Phos. and Kali. Phos. together, two tablets of each (read more about blood pressure below).

The skeleton

For aches and pains, stiff shoulders, sore back, creeping rheumatism in wet, cold weather, inflammation of muscles, joints and rheumatic pains, Ferrum Phos. is urgently indicated. Take it also for sprains, strains and stiffness. When I experience any of the above symptoms, I take two tablets every half-hour, sucked slowly until the pain is alleviated and, thereafter, three, four or even five times a day, and it can significantly ease every ache.

27

Urinary system

This tissue salt will become every woman's lifesaver. At the first hint of cystitis, two tablets each of Ferrum Phos. and Nat. Phos. should be taken every 15 minutes over a two-hour period. Nat. Phos. will make the whole urinary system more alkaline. At the same time, it is beneficial to take four teaspoons of apple cider vinegar in a glass of water, three, four or even five times during the day, to flush out the whole urinary system. When the burning sensation passes, take two tablets of Ferrum Phos. and two tablets Nat. Phos. every two to three hours for an entire day. Ferrum Phos. is essential for cases of bed-wetting (enuresis), a prolapsed uterus and bladder, a heavy sensation in the pelvis and for incontinence of urine – take two tablets four times a day.

High blood pressure

Ferrum Phos. and Kali. Phos. taken together – two tablets of each, two or three times a day – will greatly help you to feel better, in conjunction with your doctor's constant watch and medication. Don't neglect high blood pressure, don't try to treat it yourself but, with these two superb salts *as well as prescribed medication*, that desperate feeling can be significantly alleviated.

How you feel

Are you forgetful, irritable, feeling dizzy, depressed, tired or despondent? Do you have restless nights without sleep, frightening dreams, panic attacks, insomnia, and shortness of breath on exertion? If you experience feelings of being overheated and flushed, unable to cope, or generally debilitated and desperate, then the best first-aid remedy is Ferrum Phos. Take it frequently. My personal, feel-good-all-over remedy is easy to remember: tissue salts numbered 2, 4 and 6 – Calc. Phos., Ferrum Phos. and Kali. Phos. – two tablets of each three or four or five times a day – helps me with all the above symptoms even in the most dreadful circumstances. These three salts are nature's rescue remedies!

28

Secondary and complementary salts

Kali. Mur. complements Ferrum Phos. as an effective anti-inflammatory, a stimulant to the body's immune system and a normaliser of the mucous membranes, and for acute conditions and crisis conditions like sunstroke and excessive bleeding, shortness of breath and heart palpitations. Kali. Sulph. will help Ferrum Phos. improve the supply of oxygen to the tissues, as in the case of croup, and in chronic conditions like severe congestion in the nose, throat and chest. Kali. Sulph. is especially effective with Ferrum Phos. in the treatment of respiratory conditions and mucous membranes. Ferrum Phos. with Nat. Mur. is excellent for treating anaemia and, with Nat. Phos. for aching or hot, swollen joints.

Herbs that contain Ferrum Phos.

Parsley is rich in iron and should be included in the diet frequently, together with celery, horseradish, and dandelion. These four herbs all help to flush toxins out of the body, to clear infection, cleanse kidneys and bladder, acting as effective diuretics. Sesame seeds, yarrow, garlic, garlic chives and stinging nettle all have a high iron content and fight infections. They also help to clear the acid build-up that settles in the joints causing inflammatory conditions.

Foods rich in Ferrum Phos.

Spinach, lentils, radishes, onions, walnuts, strawberries, apples, lettuce – all the beautiful varieties of lettuce – also almonds, sesame seeds, leeks and garlic. Red meat and liver are also rich sources of iron and are best served grilled with lemon juice. Use stinging nettle tops (picked with gloves on) cooked with spinach and served with fresh lemon juice as a cleansing dish.

Eat at least seven of the above listed items daily to maintain good health. Kelp tablets, made from seaweed, are an important supplement as this also contains iron.

Health Booster Salad

Try this easy recipe as part of your daily menu when 'flu or cold symptoms threaten.

$^1/_2$ cup chopped celery
$^1/_2$ cup fresh chopped parsley
$^1/_2$ cup fresh chopped onions or garlic chives
$^1/_2$ cup fresh sliced radishes
$^1/_2$ cup fresh chopped spinach

$^1/_2$ to 1 cup lettuce leaves
$^1/_2$ cup chopped dandelion leaves
$^1/_2$ to 1 cup grated apple (peel removed)
$^1/_2$ cup sesame seeds sprinkled
$^1/_2$ cup chopped walnuts or almonds

the juice of 1 lemon as a salad dressing

Mix everything together and eat half for lunch and the other half for supper. Keep covered in the refrigerator. Serves 2

Health Booster Soup

A quick and easy soup recipe, this is ideal to treat all the above ailments. Serve it to anyone suffering from 'flu, bronchitis, pneumonia, or any infection, on a twice a day basis. Make a large pot, store in the refrigerator and heat a portion, as needed.

1 cup pearl barley soaked for 1 hour in hot water (or preferably overnight)
2 cups lentils
2 large onions finely chopped
1 cup onion greens or leeks
2 cups chopped celery leaves and stalks
1 cup chopped parsley
2 cups chopped lettuce green, outer leaves especially the juice of one lemon

1 cup radishes and their leaves, chopped
sea salt and black pepper to taste
2 litres of good chicken stock
a little olive oil

Fry the onions and leeks in the oil until starting to brown. Add the celery and stir-fry. Add radishes, radish leaves and continue to stir-fry. Add the remaining ingredients except parsley. Stir and cover. Simmer gently for about 1 hour. Add extra water if it becomes too thick. Adjust seasoning. Add the parsley in the last 5 minutes of cooking. Serve hot, sprinkled with sesame seeds. Serves 6–8

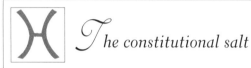

The constitutional salt

This is the tissue salt most needed by people born under the astrological sign of Pisces. The Piscean nature, like all the water signs, is often vulnerable, emotional and may suffer from scattered energies, usually with a feeling of being both exhausted physically and emotionally drained. Ferrum Phos. is a marvellous health tonic for us all, but it is particularly important to every Piscean. Take a couple of tablets daily, even twice daily, to focus on the task in hand. For indifference and listlessness and quick irritability, often found in the Pisces nature, Ferrum Phos. helps enormously. One of my children is a Piscean and, when she was still a child, I always watched out for a pale, listless, tired little face, knowing her mood could be quickly corrected with a tablet or two of Ferrum Phos. Once administered, her happy, laughing, nature would be quickly restored.

If you, or anyone in your family, suffers from any of the above symptoms, always keep Ferrum Phos. close at hand. It really is a lifesaver in every sense of the word.

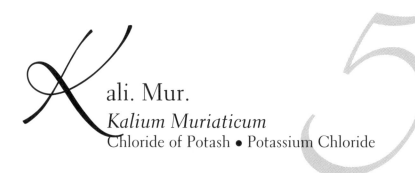

Kali. Mur.
Kalium Muriaticum
Chloride of Potash • Potassium Chloride

This tissue salt is characterised by the following functions: a decongestant, blood and lymph cleanser, waste eliminator and a second stage inflammation reducer. Subtle in its action, Kali. Mur. works very much like its cousin, Kali. Sulph. Although it may be overshadowed in its scope of ability by other salts, like Ferrum Phos. and Nat. Mur., Kali. Mur. is nevertheless just as important in its action as the other 11 tissue salts.

Potassium chloride joins with albumin to form 'fibrin', a nitrogenous protein fibre that forms part of every single body tissue, including nerves, muscles, blood – everything except the actual bones. Where there is a lack of potassium chloride (Kali. Mur.), the release of albumin will occur and, being of a thick, very cloying consistency, it is difficult to expel from the body. This discharge comes mostly from mucous membranes and occurs following an inflammatory fluid retentive stage (where Ferrum Phos. is needed). So, it could be said that Kali. Mur. is needed for the second stage of inflammation.

Dr. Schuessler believed Kali. Mur. builds fibrin and, through past decades, his theory has been proved correct. He realised brain cells cannot form without fibrin, nor can muscles or nerves. Kali. Mur. and Kali. Sulph resemble one another closely and are indicated for many of the same problems. But there is, however, one big difference between them, in that the colour of the discharge fluid requiring Kali. Mur. is white – for example nasal or bronchial catarrhs and sputum – as opposed to the yellow fluid in discharges that need Kali. Sulph. This gently working salt is often given when nothing else seems to work, particularly for chronic ailments.

The 'key' functions of Kali. Mur. are an effective decongestant, a glandular tonic, an ache reliever, a tonic for convalescents and a healer of the second stage of inflammation. Taken when a fever starts to recede, Kali. Mur. is a building agent, effectively helping the body to heal itself and recover from illness.

Ailments treated

The head
White, flaky dandruff shows a need for Kali. Mur. – but it needs to be taken over a long period. Be aware that the flakiness will increase initially, as it is clearing the waste cycle. This tissue salt is also ideal for a 'sick headache', when nausea can result from eating incorrectly or from over-indulgence. A useful combination is Kali. Mur. with Nat. Sulph. – one tablet of each sucked every 10 to 15 minutes until the condition eases. But it may result in the need to vomit sour white mucous.

The ears, eyes, nose and throat
Any evidence of thick white mucous, like crusts forming at the corner of the eyes, as a retinal discharge, even granulation on the eyelids or thick nasal catarrh show a need for Kali. Mur. That horrid cracking noise in the ears or nose and sinuses, or stuffiness in the nose, throat and chest – all are indications that Kali. Mur. is deficient. Also evident will be enlarged lymph glands in the neck and behind the ears. Tonsils and adenoids will be swollen, and possibly covered with white pustules. All these symptoms respond to two tablets of Kali. Mur. taken every 20 minutes over a period of two hours, thereafter every two to three hours until the condition clears. Remember that Kali. Mur. should be given routinely, along with Ferrum Phos. for colds and catarrh, middle-ear infection and the residue left after the fever has gone.

The mouth
Kali. Mur. is the first remedy to take if there is thrush in the mouth. I have a reliable cure for thrush that has never failed me. Anxious young mothers in the rural areas bring their fretful crying babies to

me. I keep a standard box of Kali. Mur. and a large planted area of 'sour fig' (*Carpobrotus edulis*) – that easy-to-grow succulent we use for bluebottle stings when at the beach. Use the liquid form of Kali. Mur. and give 10 drops directly into baby's mouth. Then, about 10 minutes later, using a clean finger, squeeze the juice from a 5 cm-length of the fleshy leaf of the sour fig onto the finger and rub it all over the inflamed gums and little ulcers. Repeat this several times – the succulent juice is very astringent and baby won't like it. Apply every hour for at least six hours then, suddenly, it's gone! If the mouth is very red and swollen, I alternate Kali. Mur. with Ferrum Phos. every ½ hour, both in drop form – 10 or so drops of each – into the mouth or on a clean finger and wipe over the area liberally. I give the mothers extra Kali. Mur. drops to take home and a piece of sour fig to plant near their kitchen door and they never needed to come back. They learn to give Kali. Mur. to their babies as a preventative measure whenever they see that telltale redness and swelling and the little ulcers appearing.

Digestive system and the liver

Kali. Mur. is essential for an overloaded digestive system – tired, sluggish liver and jaundice – and, when fatty foods or bread and pastries cause heartburn and sour belching. If you're eating too much white sugar, biscuits and cakes, chocolates or sweets, or suffer from digestive allergies, you're actually taxing your poor liver. Take two tablets of Kali. Mur. three to four times a day. This is about the same amount of potassium chloride that is in a naturally healthy cell.

The action on the blood by Kali. Mur. is to thin it – the reason why taking it is so important for an overloaded, sluggish liver. For a heavy drinker or an alcoholic, Kali. Mur. is vitally important (along with other salts of course) but, for the health of the liver, this important cell salt must be the first consideration.

Menstruation and female problems

With any congestion in the pelvic area, i.e. that bloated feeling, menstrual pains, dark blood clots in an excessive, dark menstrual flow, Kali. Mur. is essential. But, it must be taken in conjunction with Ferrum Phos. (to put back the iron), and Mag. Phos. (for accompanying cramps and pain relief). The overall improvement after a few doses is usually noticeable – two tablets taken frequently, dissolved under the tongue until the discomfort and congestion eases. (Incidentally, this dose is equally helpful for painful, congested haemorrhoids.) If there is any sign of a thick white discharge between menstrual cycles – known as leucorrhea – Kali. Mur. is essential. For chronic cystitis, cystic fibrosis, take Kali. Mur. in conjunction with Ferrum Phos., to gain immediately relief. Take two tablets of each three or four times a day until the symptoms subside.

Male problems
Kali. Mur. is the best cell salt to treat the prostate gland when the enlargement is soft and spongy. If the enlargement of the prostate gland is hard, then add Silica and Calc. Fluor. to ease the congestion. Two tablets of each, taken every hour for about six hours, will give relief and, thereafter, take the same dose three or four times a day until the symptoms subside.

Respiratory system
When a respiratory condition is in its 'secondary stage', for example bronchitis with much production of phlegm, or tight wheezing of asthma, croup, pneumonia or pleurisy, two Kali. Mur. tablets sucked slowly every 15 minutes will greatly alleviate the stressful condition. Similarly, in productive emphysema, when taken with Calc. Fluor., Kali. Mur. will do much to ease the discomfort. Take two tablets of each, every ½ hour to clear the passages and as a general tonic. Repeat the dose four times a day thereafter.

The joints and the skeleton
The structural bone system responds comfortingly to Kali. Mur. if there are chronic aches, such as backache, shoulder pains and stiffness, and those dull aching pains that get labelled 'rheumatism or arthritis'. And, especially when there is chronic swelling and joint pain. Even for pain experienced when resting or lying down, and that stiff frustration of a chronic back, Kali. Mur. is very soothing when taken often. Combine it with Ferrum Phos. or other appropriate salts. Lots of exercise and a diet rich in fruit and vegetables will help regain the suppleness and strength we all long for.

The skin and childhood diseases

Kali. Mur. is 'the' salt for infectious childhood diseases – chicken pox, measles, scarlet fever, even mumps – due to the swelling of the lymph glands. In cases of smallpox, chicken pox and measles, Kali. Mur. is vitally important when the activity of pustules or blisters has begun, after the fever has started to abate. When you see and understand this condition, you'll appreciate why Kali. Mur. is so important. I used this method on all my children and not one scar was ever left, thanks to Kali. Mur. It also cured much of the irritating itch. As a frequently applied *lotion* to stop the itching, dab on a solution of 30 Kali. Mur. drops in one cup of water, applied with cotton wool pads over the poxes and rash. Take two tablets of Kali. Mur. every ½ hour for at least the first day, thereafter six times a day.

The lining cells of body tissue form a thin covering (a membrane) over the cells that secrete enough moisture to keep the tissue cells healthy and nourished. But, if the membrane becomes inflamed or attacked by a virus or bacteria, the fluid-secreting ability increases in order to protect the membrane and it can become watery and copious. Nat. Mur. will ease the wateriness. Then, the next stage is the mucous, pus or fibrin formation, and Kali. Mur. will remove that 'waste' – and a build-up of mucous-catarrh too.

Weeping eczema and psoriasis can also be helped in this way. Rashes, boils and infected acne abscesses can be cleared with Kali. Mur., also cradle cap and inflamed crusty vaccinations too. Use the Kali. Mur. lotion to dissolve the crusts first.

Other general ailments

The more you use Kali. Mur. the more surprised you'll be at its diversity – diseases of the heart, including dropsy; diseases of the liver, including cirrhosis, jaundice, and after the first stages of hepatitis; whooping cough, croup and pneumonia.

This tissue salt also treats:

- peeling of the skin
- gastric fever
- feelings of weariness and heaviness of limb

- snoring
- presence of warts
- long-term lymphatic congestion
- immune system deficiency
- ongoing inflammatory stages
- recurring infection, such as recurring ear infections and a dry cough with a difficult expulsion of mucous and frequent common colds; sinusitis and headache with blocked sinuses
- raised pale patches on gums and tongue
- chronic hay fever (taken with Nat. Mur.)
- stiff hands like writer's cramp
- purulent acne
- flatulence
- itchy blisters or crusts on scalp
- minor burns
- white ulcers in the mouth
- glandular fever
- bursitis, often in the elbow or hip
- candida
- vesicular eczema

And, for the psychological (emotional) state of 'hanging on' to recycled rubbish, Kali. Mur. is a waste disposer. For someone who rehashes over and over past hurts and problems, Kali. Mur. helps to get rid of it, to metaphorically 'spit it out', like old phlegm that's been in your throat for too long!

Secondary and complementary salts

Kali. Mur. works well with Ferrum Phos. Together they tackle immune dysfunction, clearing away old problems. Remember that Ferrum Phos. is for the first stage of inflammation, Kali. Mur. for the second stage and Kali. Sulph. for the third stage. But be aware that these three stages do not necessarily follow on one after the other. They can exist all together in the body, so it's wise to take all three tissue salts.

Herbs that contain Kali. Mur.

- Violet (*Viola odorata*) – the garden violet – helps to clear mucous from the body, stops sinus build-up and clears headaches.
- Yarrow (*Achillea millefolium*) is excellent for conditions involving catarrh build-up, is a circulatory stimulant and for menstrual disorders. It helps to bring down fevers, is an excellent diuretic resolving swellings, and encourages bile flow.
- Mullein (*Verbascum thapsus*) is one of the best treatments to dissolve mucous, it can be used in cases of bronchitis, pneumonia, asthma and tuberculosis. It is also an excellent expectorant, anti-inflammatory and wound healer.
- Ginger (*Zingiber officinale*) is a superb expectorant, which promotes sweating and brings down fevers. It prevents vomiting, soothing the feeling of nausea, and relaxes peripheral blood vessels to enable wastes to be removed. It is also an effective antiseptic.
- Fennel (*Foeniculum vulgare*) is a diuretic, gently cleansing and detoxifying the system. It is a circulatory stimulant, anti-inflammatory and also a mild expectorant.
- Basil (*Ocimum basilicum*) stimulates the adrenal cortex to produce its own cortisone and soothe itching. It has antiseptic, expectorant, antidepressant and detoxifying qualities. Use fresh in salads.
- Borage (*Borago officinalis*) relieves eczema, regulates menstruation, is an adrenal stimulant, an expectorant, promotes sweating and is an anti-rheumatic.
- Sage (*Salvia officinalis* only) has antiseptic and natural antibiotic qualities, promotes bile flow, reduces blood sugar, and is an antispasmodic. It is excellent for respiratory ailments and treats sore throats, coughs, colds and 'flu.

Make a *tea* with ¼ cup fresh leaves to one cup boiling water. Stand five minutes and strain. Take one to two cups daily until the condition clears.

Foods rich in Kali. Mur.

Green beans, carrots, beetroot, squash, cauliflower, kale, green mealies and mealie meal porridge, asparagus, celery, peaches, apricots, pineapples, lemons and plums are all sources of this mineral salt. Eat at least eight of these fruits and vegetables daily.

The constitutional tissue salt

Kali. Mur. is most needed by those born under the astrological sign of Gemini as they have a vitality that's more on the mental level than the physical and they can easily burn out. The Gemini personality is quick, alert, and impatient, rapidly changing in thought, mood and perception, which tends to create over-stimulation. This huge scattering of nervous energy means Kali. Mur. is a daily and absolute necessity. Two tablets taken twice to six times a day will help Gemini to structure, to plan and to wind down.

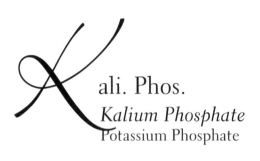

ali. Phos.
Kalium Phosphate
Potassium Phosphate

Kali. Phos. is characterised by the following functions: a brain and nerve tonic and a nerve nutrient. It promotes a feeling of well-being as it calms, uplifts and, as such, is a constituent of all the fluids in the body. In a nutshell, Kali. Phos. helps to relieve the day-to-day pressures caused by tension, stress and jangled nerves – it helps you to cope and keep calm.

With an antiseptic action, Kali. Phos. is one of the most unusual salts in its performance of slowing down or stopping the decay of body tissue. This is applicable in, for example, paralysis or nerve degeneration. It is also beneficial in cases where there is a deficient nerve supply to a part of the body with restricted mobility.

Sufferers of depression, insomnia, nervous tension, a nervous breakdown or hyper-sensitivity will all find Kali. Phos. helpful. This tissue salt is currently and increasingly being tested and considered for the treatment of excessive hyperactivity, for autism, for suicidal tendencies and for dyslexia. So think about adding this tissue salt as your daily remedy.

Ailments treated

The emotional mind
Kali. Phos. is one of the most important tissue salts for the over-emotional and for the mental symptoms of worry and distress. For that feeling of anticipatory anxiety or dread, butterflies in the stomach and the mind being confused and indecisive with over-stimulation and worry, Kali. Phos. is the answer: two tablets

under the tongue taken every 10-20 minutes will lift and lighten the mood. When there is mental fatigue, burnout and loss of memory, particularly for students during exam times, Kali. Phos. will stimulate the brain. Take it in conjunction with Mag. Phos. for prolonged stress or burnout, and total exhaustion.

Be aware that the typical personality who really needs to take Kali. Phos. will exhibit the following reclusive traits: they will not want to go out or enjoy the prospect of any social event, they will avoid being part of any demanding situation. And, I watch myself here carefully, for the moment everything gets to be too much and I cannot bear to leave my farm, I immediately top up on Kali. Phos. – two tablets taken six times a day – and next day I'm back to normal and can take on the world!

A natural tranquilliser

It's all too easy to take a prescription drug but it is far, far safer to fight every depression naturally. To calm irritable tempers, to banish worry, diminish symptoms of overwork, over-excitement or over-anxiety – in every case where a tranquilliser is needed – Kali. Phos. is the answer.

I often combine it with Calc. Phos. four to six times a day (two tablets of each), for as long as the symptoms persist. Kali. Phos. is the natural 'pick-me-up' tonic. Use it in times of grief or sorrow, disappointment, despair, a broken love affair, and those times when you awaken crying inconsolably in the night.

Kali. Phos. will help to raise one's mood during times of absolute desperation, heart-sore occasions when someone you love is dying, or has passed away. It should be taken when life is wearying and joyless, when direction to life has been lost and particularly for those people who suffer from panic attacks. Kali. Phos., two tablets taken frequently, is a sure remedy!

Do you dread noise? Does the barking of neighbours' dogs, loud music, children's yells and screams, traffic sounds, aircraft – all the noise pollution that humanity creates – drive you mad? Then Kali. Phos. is your calming, soothing tranquilliser. And it is also ideal for those exhausting hyperactive children – both for you and for them!

Does your memory play tricks and you become forgetful, or suffer from poor concentration? Or perhaps your vitality flags and you are beset with melancholy moods. If the change-of-life despondency is part of every day, and when you feel you cannot cope and feel weepy, or sleepwalk or are obsessed with nightmares and you don't know what to do – take Kali. Phos. – two tablets under the tongue – up to 10 times a day. Many elderly folk develop a fear of dying or suffer symptoms of senility. Both of which can be alleviated by taking this cell salt. And, if you recognise the heavy-hearted, tired-of-life, afraid-of-death mentality, then Kali. Phos. is the salt for you!

The head
For that blinding ache at the back of the head, with dizziness or confusion, Kali. Phos. – two tablets under the tongue every 10 minutes – will help steady you. For epilepsy, exhaustion and inability to think, or a nervous headache from loss of sleep or too much work, Kali. Phos. should be taken with Mag. Phos. – two tablets of each every 10 minutes. And this remedy will also soothe a pain over the eyes or neuralgia pains.

There is evidence that Kali. Phos. is extremely helpful in treating Bell's palsy, where a sudden infection in facial nerves causes paralysis to one side of the face. It is also beneficial in treating a stroke – CVA or a cerebral vascular accident. Two tablets of Kali. Phos. taken every hour for the first 10 or so hours, thereafter four to six times a day, will result in a steady improvement.

The eyes and ears
In cases where blurred or weakening vision is experienced, or if flashes of colour appear before the eyes or in the periphery vision, two tablets of Kali. Phos., taken four to six times a day will help to clear the problem. The same dose applies to treating other distortions in vision, such as a 'halo' effects, and those worrisome floating black spots, or astigmatism, a dry sensation in the eyes or glaucoma.

If eye fatigue is suffered as a result of staring at a computer screen for many hours, take two tables of Kali. Phos. four to six times a day. The same dose applies to exhaustion of the optic nerve or red, bloodshot and aching eyes from studying in poor light accompanied by twitches at the corner of the eye.

To treat that roaring, buzzing sounds in the ears, and if the ears are swollen, pulsating, or even twitching, two tablets of Kali. Phos. taken every 15 minutes, will help.

Ageing

'Old age surely isn't for sissies,' as someone aptly observed, and, as my eighty-seven-year-old mother says: 'Old age has nothing to recommend it!' But she takes her tissue salts consistently and walks at a great pace round her locality, takes an active interest in politics, and looks 70. One day I hope to emulate her. She finds the tissue salts 'get rid of all those beastly little problems that so often trip you up'.

Kali. Phos. is helpful for all the worries related to ageing in the elderly – such as a fear of becoming ill, incontinence, bed sores, financial problems, blurred vision, insomnia and the remorse that tend to engulf one. And don't forget that weak feeling in the extremities. Another worry is the inability to concentrate, and those frightening night terrors. Losing one's mental faculty and abilities, (senility and Alzheimer's disease) is very distressing. So too is loss of vitality and energy allied to withdrawing from people and becoming reclusive. Bad moods, tearfulness, irritability, poor memory and a great suspicion of other people's activities and motives often accompany this mental deterioration. For all these ailments two tablets of Kali. Phos. should be taken twice or three times a day in conjunction with Silica (two tablets twice or three times a day) and watch the improvement.

When there is a lack of Kali. Phos. in the motor nerves, there will be a weakness in nerve response and corresponding weak muscle action, sometimes with paralysis or with pain and a sensation of numbness. Take two tablets of Kali. Phos. three times a day or more.

Digestive system

A lack or deficiency of Kali. Phos. characteristically shows itself as a craving for food, even directly after a large meal. It is almost a feeling of exhaustion from not eating or lack of food, in spite of the stomach being full. It also eliminates a bitter taste in the mouth and chattering teeth.

Butterflies in the stomach before an event can be quelled with Kali. Phos., as can indigestion and flatulence, if the food has been taken at a time when one was upset, frightened or worried – all symptoms of nervous indigestion or dyspepsia.

Remember that Kali. Phos. is an extremely important element in the process of metabolism, as well as in the digestion of fats. Kali. Phos. is a cleanser of all putrefactive conditions like an overloaded gassy bowel, bad-smelling diarrhoea and acute infections of the gastric tract. Symptoms like gastritis, gastro-enteritis and inflammation of the colon will all benefit from Kali. Phos., two tablets taken four to six times throughout the day.

Circulatory system
It is rare to find any case histories on high blood pressure, but there is excellent evidence that Kali. Phos., taken in conjunction with Ferrum Phos., three to five times a day (two tablets of each with your doctor's prescribed medication) will make you feel better.

Note: Never attempt to treat yourself for high blood pressure – always consult your doctor and have it checked weekly.

If there is slow or insufficient flow of blood to the brain, when dizziness, vertigo, faintness can be experienced, take two tablets each of Kali. Phos. combined with Mag. Phos., every 10 minutes until the condition clears. The same treatment will alleviate heart palpitations and nervous upsets that cause palpitations or an irregular heart beat. It also helps for emotional tensions that cause an irregular heart beat and in cases of poor immunity and injuries where septic conditions develop.

Respiratory system
This is one of the most comforting uses for this tissue salt – treating nervous asthma, tight coughs, obstructed swollen nose, allergic hay fever, childhood asthma, and even for a long-term cough and chronic asthma. Again, when Kali. Phos. is taken with Mag. Phos., the distressing symptoms will quickly respond and bring breathing and discomfort back to normal. That over-stimulated nervous system that results in frightened, wheezing and asthmatic spasm and short, gasping breaths will be alleviated.

Take two tablets of each every 10 minutes until a state of calmness and easy breathing is reached.

Female problems
Take Kali. Phos. to ease painful period pains and, by the way, it is a lifesaver for the famous PMT (premenstrual tension). This topic regularly appears in women's magazines, where each article gives complicated advice on how to deal with it – when Kali. Phos. does the trick so quickly and so easily! Take two tablets three times a day with Mag. Phos. Start taking the tablets three days before the period is due and carry on right through. Remember it when that lassitude and the heavy mood swings mark this time of the month.

For pregnancy problems, Kali. Phos. is wonderful and especially for protracted labour when it is necessary to increase vitality when the need to push comes!

Male problems
Kali. Phos. is now found to be a great help for impotence, particularly if it follows prolonged mental fatigue, stress and burnout. Also if there is a strong sexual desire but reduced potency, two tablets three to six times a day has proved to be helpful.

Skin problems
I am often asked to advise with the incidence of eczema or itchy rashes that appear during times of stress or anxiety, also stress-related hair loss (alopecia) or the involuntary pulling out or excessive fiddling with and tugging and twisting of one's hair. All these complaints will respond to two tablets of Kali. Phos. taken four times a day. Shingles is an exceptionally painful ailment. The skin is excessively tender over the affected area and it is difficult to get relief from the discomfort, but Kali. Phos. with Mag. Phos. will help. Two tablets of each taken every half an hour will help a sufferer through the most trying time, and thereafter four times a day until the condition clears.

Some specific illnesses
This list is an unusual one, but use of Kali. Phos. is so important I have given each its own space.

45

Yuppie 'flu

In recent years, one of the most intensively debilitating illnesses has been yuppie 'flu (Guillain-Barré syndrome), with an array of weakening peculiarities. And here, Kali. Phos. is particularly helpful when taken six to 10 times throughout the day. Potassium acts as a detergent in the bowel and in fact in the whole digestive system, and it is vital to the health, the ability and the action of the heart.

Cancer

Some doctors are seriously considering potassium's chemical action as a protective, preventative factor in cancer. Certain European doctors, including my old Swiss doctor who loved tissue salts so sincerely, believe some cancers are caused by a potassium imbalance, and this is why they prescribe Kali. Phos., as it is so easily assimilated. Apart from recommending a diet of potassium-rich foods, these doctors also suggest a drastic reduction in the intake of table salt.

Brainpower

In this unique biochemical preparation, potassium is mixed carefully with phosphoric acid until it becomes slightly more alkaline (as opposed to acid). It is also important to point out that this substance is vital to brain chemistry, as it can combine so well with other vital substances to form grey matter.

Angina pectoris

Another important contribution Kali. Phos. can make is in the case of angina pectoris, but only in association with the doctor's advice and treatment. The actual physiology of angina can be eased by frequently taking Kali. Phos. with Mag. Phos.

It is important to remember that everything to do with the heart can be helped by Kali. Phos. and Mag. Phos. – but only in conjunction with what medication your doctor prescribes. For fat around the heart, for pain in the chest, inflamed lungs, Kali. Phos. with Mag. Phos. is often a lifesaver.

46

Excessive body odour

An embarrassing ailment is offensive body odour. But, in conjunction with Silica and Nat. Phos., Kali. Phos. is tremendously helpful. Two tablets of each taken four times a day for two to three months will generally clear the personal odour problem completely. One lady, suffering from this embarrassing complaint, took the three tissue salts for 10 days and the odour disappeared. And she even mentioned to me that her son's extra smelly feet are 'smelling like a rose' since he also took the three cell salts.

Gangrene

For gangrene – where there is little nerve supply and circulation to a part of the body – Kali. Phos. is vitally important. Use it as a lotion to massage into the parts as well, provided the skin is unbroken – add 20 drops of Kali. Phos. to one litre of warm water. Take two tablets of Kali. Phos. and two tablets of Ferrum Phos. up to 10 times a day and massage all around the affected area. As a physiotherapist, I treated many cases with much success. Ask your doctor to consider this.

Secondary and complementary salts

As described above, Mag. Phos. enhances and complements Kali. Phos., due to the analgesic action, but Kali. Phos. and Calc. Phos. share their abilities to tone the body. Calc. Phos. is taken where there is no elasticity in the structure of the tissues, and Kali. Phos. is essential where there is no tone, because the nerve supply to the tissues is absent or partially lacking. Ferrum Phos. is another helpful partner to Kali. Phos. for improved circulation to an area of the body.

Herbs that contain Kali. Phos.

- St. John's Wort: rich in phosphorus and potassium, it is an astringent, an analgesic, anti-inflammatory, a sedative and, wait for it, a restorative tonic to the nervous system!
- Ginger: excellent for high blood pressure, it stimulates the circulation and is generally useful for arteriosclerosis, for digestive disturbances,

nausea and travel sickness. A comforting treatment for coughs, colds and asthma, it is also an antiseptic and anti-inflammatory.

- Mustard: a circulatory and digestive stimulant and a diuretic, mustard stimulates the gastric juices and therefore aids digestion.
- Horseradish: another stimulating herb like ginger and mustard, horseradish aids circulation and digestion, is a powerful antibacterial and has cancer protective qualities. It is a wonderful remedy for coughs, 'flu, colds, sinus problems, and one that makes you really feel better as it stimulates the endorphins.
- Red clover: one of the important anti-cancer herbs, it is antispasmodic, diuretic, anti-inflammatory, and is good for arthritic and wandering pains, respiratory ailments and treats eczema and psoriasis.
- Thyme: a wonderful antiseptic, an expectorant and an excellent skin herb, thyme is also widely used for treating bronchitis and other respiratory problems. A natural antibiotic, it heals wounds and increases the blood flow to an area.
- Chives and garlic: both contain natural antibiotic and anti-coagulant substances and they (particularly garlic) are effective expectorants, they reduce blood cholesterol and blood sugar levels while boosting the immune system.

Foods rich in Kali. Phos.

Lettuce and all green, leafy vegetables like spinach, beetroot tops, amaranth, radish leaves as well as the actual radish, olives, oats, green mustard leaves, onions, garlic, walnuts, cauliflower, broccoli, green beans, lentils, potatoes, tomatoes, lemons, guavas, cherries, apples and dates are all rich in Kali. Phos.

Eat at least seven items from this list daily, for any of the Kali. Phos. indications described above. It is so worth growing your own vegetables and fruits organically. I plant a 'Kali. Phos. greens' garden every season, using summer vegetables and winter ones to keep fit and happy. It is also worth growing a precious lemon tree (Meyer lemons do well in pots) and if you live in a frost free area, a guava tree, and an apple or walnut tree for colder areas. This way you can harvest your own health giving fruits and vegetables.

48

Kali. Phos. fruit salad

This is a quick and easy pick-me-up, especially during exam times, to boost brainpower.

4 apples, peeled and coarsely grated

½ cup fresh raw ginger, grated

½ cup dates, finely chopped

3 cups fresh ripe guavas, peeled and coarsely grated or chop finely if flesh is very soft

2 cups fresh cherries, stoned (if in season)

2 cups paw-paw, peeled and diced

Mix everything together well in a glass bowl. Then mix 2 tablespoons honey with 2 tablespoons lemon juice and pour over. Serve chilled with a little plain yogurt. Serves 4

 ## The constitutional tissue salt

Kali. Phos. is the tissue salt most needed by people born under the astrological sign of Aries. For mental burnout, physical exhaustion, the relentless activity and nervous anxiety that frequently engulfs Aries, Kali. Phos. is a serious need. For depression and behaviour problems allied to hypersensitivity – so much a part of being Aries – take two tablets of Kali. Phos. daily, as part of your 'must have' schedule. Neglect it and you'll pay the price.

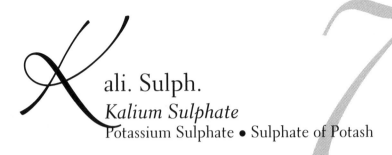

Kali. Sulph.
Kalium Sulphate
Potassium Sulphate • Sulphate of Potash

Kali. Sulph. is an effective distributor of oxygen. In the same way that Ferrum Phos. regulates the 'external breathing' of the cells, so Kali. Sulph. provides the same internal function of the cells in the exchange of oxygen for carbon dioxide. This tissue salt helps to keep the membrane tissue healthy, and it treats the third level of an infection or inflammation. This is the development stage of the infection when an antibiotic is usually prescribed in conventional medicine (as in thick mucous blocking the nose, ears and bronchi in the process of a dose of 'flu or bronchitis). It is important to realise that it is at this stage of the infection when Kali. Sulph. is able to carry oxygen to the cells, thus assisting the healing action.

Although its effects are not as dramatic as those of other cell salts Kali. Sulph. has the ability to achieve unique results that combine well with other salts. Dr. Schuessler's belief maintains that the active ingredients in many botanical remedies are actually the 12 tissue salts, and this theory is clearly evident in Kali. Sulph., yet it can easily be overlooked. I have in the past noted some chronic ailments that were cured by Kali. Sulph. – cases where the medical world had given up, just a few doses taken daily over one or two months can change people's lives.

Ailments treated

The skin
This tissue salt has a close connection to the lining cells of the skin and to the internal mucous membranes of all body organs. If there is a

disturbance in these lining cells, a discharge occurs – either flaky, dry cells or a yellowish, slimy matter. Kali. Sulph., together with the oxygen in the body, activates the removal of worn-out cells. It normalises and cleanses and, to my mind, this ability makes it a very important skin salt – it helps to build new cells! Kali. Sulph. is essential in the treatment of psoriasis, eczema, and itchy dry skin on the hands and feet, rashes, warts and, on the scalp, ringworm, flaky dry patches, dandruff and baldness. It also helps heal eruptions such as herpes blisters, pimples, rough, red skin and fungal attacks. Where old skin cells have been damaged due to disease, Kali. Sulph. repairs. Before considering a facelift, try Kali. Sulph. first – it is a skin rejuvenator!

For children suffering with eczema and rashes or childhood diseases, such as chicken pox or measles, give Kali. Sulph. in liquid form. It works well and can be used as a *lotion* – dilute 20 drops in ½ cup of warm water and dab on or spray the affected area. (Treat all childhood diseases with Kali. Sulph. to assist in the formation of new skin cells.) The liquid form of Kali. Sulph. is useful for adults too. Use it for lightening and clearing liver or age spots, freckles, scaly eruptions on moist skin and also for treating shaving rash. Spray or dab on the lotion (as described above) three times a day. As a skin lubricator, Kali. Sulph. helps to keep the skin supple and youthful. For all the conditions mentioned above take two tablets of Kali. Sulph. three to five times a day until the condition clears, and thereafter twice a day.

The eyes

If there is poor or failing vision or visual disturbances, Kali. Sulph. will help. The same applies if eyelids become itchy, red or swollen and there is inflammation of the conjunctiva – often accompanied by a crusty discharge in the corners of the eyes. Take two tablets of Kali. Sulph. three times a day to clear or greatly alleviate these symptoms.

The head

When there is congestion, thick sinuses, blocked nose and a sinus headache or one caused by a hot stuffy room, take Kali. Sulph. It is also recommended to treat falling hair, lifeless, dull, straggly hair and sticky dandruff, flakiness and serious alopecia (hair loss). In the latter cases, this tissue salt is urgently needed. Kali. Sulph. also helps to clear that thick fuzzy feeling when thinking is muddled or unclear. Take two tablets of Kali. Sulph. three to four times a day until the conditions clears, thereafter once or twice a day.

The ears
In cases where deafness is due to chronic catarrh, blocked ears, a thick yellow discharge or dark wax accompanied by consistent earache, take Kali. Sulph. In the case of children, particularly, with a residual cough and congestion in their ears, nose and throat, Kali. Sulph. will ease the problem. Two tablets taken four to six times a day will greatly alleviate all these congested conditions, and, for small children 10 to 20 drops in ½ a glass of water, taken two to four times a day will quickly restore health.

Respiratory system
For all sorts of chest infections, from bronchitis and pneumonia in the third or later stage, to a chronic cough and asthma, two tablets of Kali. Sulph. four to eight times a day will start clearing the problem. Dr. Schuessler prescribed lots of Kali. Sulph. during a feverish cold as it also promotes perspiration, thus reducing the temperature. And, it should also be taken, as mentioned above, for whooping cough to relieve the spasm.

Digestive system
A thick yellowish coating on the tongue – especially at the back of the tongue – is a sure indication that Kali. Sulph. is lacking. This tissue salt, in conjunction with Mag. Phos., also helps to allay sugar cravings. It also relieves the uncomfortable feeling of fullness in the gut, accompanied with sulphur-smelling flatulence and yellow diarrhoea or a thin black stool. These symptoms are often accompanied by an intense anal itch and haemorrhoids, or colic or a burning pain in the lower part of the bowel. Taking two tablets of Kali. Sulph. every 15 minutes until the condition eases can relieve all these uncomfortable and distressing symptoms.

Female problems

For cooling those nasty hot flushes associated with menopause, Kali. Sulph. definitely helps, and, especially when hot, stuffy rooms aggravate the condition, or during the oppressive heat experienced during summer. Take two tablets up to eight times a day and, for scanty, suppressed menstruation, take two tablets three times a day until your cycle becomes regular. In cases of chronic cystitis, where there is a yellow discharge – remember this is the third stage of inflammation – Kali. Sulph. is needed, two tablets four to six times a day. For backache during menstruation, two tablets three or four times a day is extremely helpful.

The nails

Kali. Sulph. is helpful in treating fungal problems in the nail bed and, incidentally, it treats skin fungus as well – for example between the toes where constant damp provides the perfect spot for fungal infestation. It is also effective where there is a thickening and distorted growth in the nail, as well as flaking and peeling. To treat any of the above problems, take two tablets of Kali. Sulph. four times a day for about 10 days, thereafter twice a day until the condition clears. At the at the same time use the liquid form of Kali. Sulph. (available from your local pharmacy) and make a *topical lotion* made by mixing 10 drops of Kali. Sulph. diluted in four tablespoons of water. Dab this on frequently. Don't forget to also use tea tree oil, dabbed onto the affected area as well.

Loss of both sense of smell and sense of taste

Three specific cell salts will help to resolve this condition: Kali. Sulph., Nat. Mur. and Nat. Sulph. Take two tablets of each four to six times a day until the condition improves, thereafter two tablets of each twice a day.

Joint pains

Rheumatic or shifting wandering pains, aching joints, stiff aching shoulders, even neuralgia of the face and jaw can be alleviated by combining Kali. Sulph. with Mag. Phos. – two tablets of each taken up to 10 times a day. Also, if you awake around 3 a.m. with aches and pains, two tablets of Kali. Sulph. taken with warm milk will help to get you back to sleep.

Other ailments

In their long list of symptoms that could be helped by Kali. Sulph., Drs. Carey and Perry included all the above-mentioned complaints. But they also highlighted critical illnesses like typhoid, typhus, fungoid inflammation of the joints, blood poisoning, small pox, deafness from swelling of the internal ear, and a feeling of suffocation. They also urge the use of Kali. Sulph., in both pill and liquid form. Apply the lotion to cancer of the face, the nose or in any part of the body. Remember to take it when that dose of 'flu progresses into bronchitis and pneumonia, and when the throat feels so tight you almost gag and find it difficult to swallow. Kali. Sulph. and Ferrum Phos. – two tablets of each dissolved in warm water sipped every 20 minutes – will quickly ease a panicky situation.

Cancer

Dr. Forbes-Ross was one of a dedicated team of doctors who believed that a shortage of potassium was one of the main causes of cancer. They offered many case histories, and suggested black molasses should be added to the diet to help assimilate a good supply of potassium into the diet. Their formula was Kali. Mur., Kali. Phos., Kali. Sulph., and Ferrum Phos. – two tablets of each to be taken four to six times a day and up to 10 times a day in severe cases, and, two tablets of each once a day as a preventative measure. Dr. Perry suggested Kali. Sulph. and Calc. Sulph. to be taken daily, two tablets of each, to protect against cancer. Kali. Sulph. has proved to be a lifesaver in many instances.

Drs. Carey and Perry also recommend consulting a physician to include injections of Kali. Sulph. and Ferrum Phos. frequently for intestinal, uterine and vaginal cancer. The dosage for any severe illness needs to be monitored by a doctor. The usual dose is two tablets of both Ferrum Phos. and Kali. Sulph. six to eight times a day.

Secondary and complementary salts

Ferrum Phos. and Kali. Sulph. are excellent together, as they strengthen and improve the respiratory tract, enabling it to expel deposits of old mucous. The action of Kali. Sulph., for the third stage of inflammation or infection, works well with Ferrum Phos. and Kali. Mur., as the latter are active (respectively) for the first and second infection stages. Often all three can be taken together as their combined action boosts the healing process. Kali. Sulph. and Calc. Sulph. also go together well as they both work on conditions that create a discharge.

Herbs that contain Kali. Sulph.

- Melissa: a soothing, calming herb that relaxes the peripheral blood vessels. It is a relaxing restorative to the nervous system and an antiviral, antibacterial and an antispasmodic.
- Watercress: rich in vitamins A, B1, B2, C and E, iron, phosphorus and potassium and an excellent detoxifying herb that helps to clear mucous production in chronic bronchitis. It is stimulating, and is a powerful diuretic.
- Parsley: a wonderful detoxifier and diuretic, it clears old infections, and cleanses the liver, lungs and kidneys while flushing out the urinary system. It also dissolves mucous. Parsley is a fabulous health food rich in minerals and vitamins.
- Salad burnet: a cleanser, diuretic and antibacterial, it clears toxins, particularly in the liver. It is rich in minerals, especially potassium.
- Linseed: use either the sprouts that are so easy to grow, or just the soaked linseed. It has excellent mineral content and also contains vitamins A, B, C and E. It is a superb antiseptic, anti-rheumatic, a diuretic, a natural laxative and it also breaks down mucous build-up.
- Mustard: sprout the seeds or eat the green leaves, or both. Rich in minerals, it breaks down mucous, detoxifies while clearing infections and boosting the circulation.

H̸ealth Salad

Combine together in a salad bowl:

1 cup of salad burnet leaves

½ cup parsley, finely chopped

2 cups of watercress

1 cup of mustard (sprouts or green leaves)

1 cup of linseed sprouts

Cover with a dressing of fresh lemon juice and eat a generous portion daily as a health boost.

Foods rich in Kali. Sulph.

The diet plays a huge role when it is vital to clear out and revitalise the whole body. Eat as many of the following foods as possible on a daily basis: fresh carrots, plain Bulgarian or Greek yoghurt, barley water (boil 1 cup of pearl barley in 2 litres of water. Simmer gently and top up water frequently for about 40 minutes. Cool then strain. Drink 1-2 glasses daily with lemon and honey to clear mucous and toxins), oats in muesli or porridge (not the instant kind), lettuce, endives, chicory, cottage cheese, almonds, rye and wholewheat bread.

 ## *T̸he constitutional tissue salt*

This is the tissue salt most needed by people born under the astrological sign of Virgo. They often exhibit irritable or overly impatient traits and tend to be over-meticulous. Kali. Sulph. – just two tablets daily – will help with many of the problems that tend to plague people born under this sign. The digestive functions of the bowel and liver are sensitive. These organs can suffer – causing lack of health and vitality – due to anxiety and irritability that can deplete the nervous system and delay the healing processes. As a result, the body can suffer prolonged illness. Kali. Sulph. is an effective cell salt to promote recuperation.

ag. Phos.
Magnesium Phosphate
Magnesium Phosphoricum • Phosphate
of Magnesia

A tissue salt with far-reaching curative abilities, Mag. Phos. is closely allied to two other phosphates, Calc. Phos. and Kali. Phos., and all three are excellent for treating pain-causing ailments of the nerves. As a natural painkiller, Mag. Phos. is also vitally important and unique.

Mag. Phos. is characterised by the following functions: it is an antispasmodic, a general painkiller and a nerve and muscle relaxant. It is found in the blood cells of bones, the teeth, the brain and the nerves and muscles. If this salt is in any way out of balance within the body, spasm and cramp will result.

Indicated to alleviate pain, Mag. Phos. should be taken for sharp constricting pains in earache, toothache and headaches, particularly. It proved effective in one of my own most spectacular personal needs – an instance when I experienced an intense all-over-the-body-itch that made me feel frantic. Two tablets taken every 10 minutes cleared it up in 18 minutes. Also, on another level of personal experience as a writer, I have the greatest respect for Mag. Phos. as I laboriously write all my books and magazine articles in longhand and Mag. Phos. clears my writer's cramp!

One of the most worrying and irritating problems is the uncontrollable shaking of the hands and, as a result, being unable to write or do the fine motor movements. Mag. Phos. becomes a great support to relieve this condition, and two tablets four to six times a day will bring much needed calm.

The words 'St. Vitus dance' have an ominous ring, but convulsions and spastic-type rigors all comfortingly respond to Mag. Phos. I am surprised and disappointed that it is not more frequently prescribed by doctors. Mag. Phos. is the main tissue salt that effects the function of the motor nerves. It is important to take it for problems like spasmodic cramps, pain during childbirth, convulsions, palpitations of the heart, consistent yawning, shivering and shaking, for unsteady handwriting and to soothe teething babies who cry with colic and flatulence. It is a spectacular tissue salt in its immediate effect. Dr. Schuessler found it extraordinarily effective for continual hiccups and also for squinting.

Ailments treated

The head

Taking Mag. Phos. can help those sharp neuralgic headaches, or stabbing pain over one eye. It is also effective for headaches induced by nervous tension and the feeling of a tight band around the head. Mag. Phos. helps to harden dental enamel and acts well to relieve toothache – especially for teeth that send stabbing pains. It also works for facial neuralgia that is sensitive when touched. Try an experiment using a warm application such as a face cloth wrung out in hot water to which several drops of liquid Mag. Phos. have been added. Hold the cloth over the area and, if this brings instant relief, then you'll know Mag. Phos. is needed. Take two tablets every 10-20 minutes until the pain or spasm recedes. Mag. Phos. is also important for tetanus (lockjaw), taken in conjunction with specified treatment by a doctor.

The eyes

If Mag. Phos. is deficient in the body, there may be disturbances which affect the vision – sparks, flashes, colours before the eyes or blurred vision of the type usually associated with a migraine attack. Similarly, muscular tension, like squinting, can also cause headaches and even abnormal dilation or constriction of the pupils or over-sensitivity to bright light. Mag. Phos. can help to obviate all these unpleasant symptoms. The usual dose is two tablets every 10-20 minutes until the condition eases. If you sometimes experience a twitching eyelid or a spasmodic winking or a fluttering tic around the eye, these nerve-related complaints can be corrected by taking Mag. Phos. – even neuralgia around the eyes will respond to this tissue salt.

The ears

Mag. Phos. is particularly helpful for ringing in the ears or pains around the ears. It also relieves earache inside the ears, otitis media, and it is one of the important remedies for treating deafness that comes with anxiety and extreme nervous tension.

Digestive system

Mag. Phos. gives quick relief for heartburn, flatulence, colic and nausea, and it also helps to quell hunger pains. Lack of magnesium has been connected with intestinal malabsorption, severe diarrhoea, bowel and stomach cramps and chronic liver disease – possibly caused by alcoholism. It is also recommended for irritable bowel syndrome, spastic colon and bloated colic.

According to Dr. John Miller, magnesium (and especially chelated magnesium) acts as a stimulant in the creation and development of enzymes that are essential to process our food. Magnesium helps to keep the blood alkaline, so the digestive process is kept normal and healthy when there is plenty available in the intestines.

Crops need magnesium too

Every farmer and vegetable grower knows how valuable magnesium is in the soil. A lack of this mineral will cause crops, especially root vegetables, to be malformed or misshapen. This deficiency is easily corrected.

As an avid vegetable grower, I had my first vegetable patch at the age of five and, among foods, vegetables and fruits are my first love. So, ever since and wherever I have lived, I have always had a vegetable garden and am quite good at keeping it organically healthy. Imagine my distress when I produced a crop of misshapen carrots and, in the next row, were blemished small and odd-shaped sweet potatoes. At the time I was unaware this indicated a magnesium deficiency. The next season, with extra compost and magnesium added to the soil, there was a magnificent crop of potatoes and carrots, and, by the way, the best green peppers, radishes and turnips I'd ever seen! Just as magnesium works beneficially in the human body, it works for vegetables too, and, as a bonus, no one experienced indigestion whatsoever from eating my exquisite green peppers and turnips – even amongst the most picky eaters!

Respiratory system

Mag. Phos. is the prime remedy for that horrid constricting feeling of the throat that sometimes affects people of a nervous disposition. It also works for any mucous membrane or bronchial spasm. Use it in conjunction with Kali. Mur. for croup, asthma and those embarrassing hiccup attacks. Take two tablets of each every 10 minutes or 10 drops of each in ½ cup warm water. It is also effective for loss of the sense of smell (but not if catarrh is involved), taken with Kali. Phos. – two tablets of each taken six times a day may help to regain the normal sense of smell.

Urinary system

For painful urination, retention of urine or nervous, spasmodic urine retention, also bed-wetting in children, Mag. Phos. is highly recommended. Adults should take two tablets up to 10 times a day. Children should be given one tablet three times during the afternoon and two before going to bed. This dose will often ease the anxiety and prevent bed-wetting. In cases of bladder stones, Mag. Phos. is essential as it eases the associated pain and spasm and, by taking Silica as well, both salts will together assist in breaking down the stones.

Female problems

Mag. Phos. is excellent for alleviating menstrual cramps, pre-menstrual pain and the tension and moodiness that accompany these symptoms. When the cramps are severe, Mag. Phos. is needed not only to ease the constriction of blood vessels but also to ease the pains associated with ovulation. Mag. Phos. is a comforting cell salt to take if there are false labour pains during pregnancy, or hot flushes during menopause but be sure to ask and follow your doctor's advice.

Male problems

Mag. Phos. is one of the best remedies for tension related to sexual problems. When one is aware that spasm and tension indicate a lack of magnesium in the body, it is easy to rectify the problem. Mag. Phos. will also help alleviate the frequent urge to urinate and pains and hypertrophy in the prostate gland. Take two tablets every ½ hour until the problem eases, thereafter two tablets twice a day.

Other ailments

Following is a rather extraordinary list I gradually compiled over the years. It has been invaluable during my years of isolation on a distant farm, bringing up my children and treating the staff and farm animals, all of which responded well to tissue salts. Mag. Phos. is the first cell salt I reach for in emergency, for any pain or spasm. And, the quickest way to ease the situation is to dissolve six tablets, or 20 drops, in ½ glass warm water, and sip it slowly.

Mag. Phos. can be used to treat a very diverse range of complaints and ailments that are grouped below into similar conditions:

- For insect bites, stings from wasps, bees or scorpions, infected mosquito bites – treat with a lotion of Mag. Phos., applied by soaking a cotton wool pad in the above solution and dab it on frequently.
- In cases of extreme exhaustion or sunstroke, for limb jerking, Parkinson's disease, and restless sleep, nightmares and night terrors, Mag. Phos. will help. It also treats sweating caused by fearfulness, muscle twitching, cold sweats, violent nausea and vomiting, severe cramps, tremors and Tourette's syndrome.
- This tissue salt even helps those folk addicted to alcohol and others suffering from the distressing results of personality changes – especially with unreasonable moods and outbursts and temper tantrums. Also, it should be taken in cases of confusion of thought, mood swings, irregular heart beat and poor sleep patterns.
- Mag. Phos. is also recommended for angina and chest pains. Call the doctor immediately, and take two tablets under the tongue straight away. Follow with two more tablets every few minutes.
- This tissue salt is also used to treat late onset diabetic ailments and tensions, spasmodic coughing and breathlessness, convulsions, sciatica nerve pains down the leg and associated lower back pain.
- It helps in the digestive system for colic and diarrhoea.
- Mag. Phos. can even be taken for cramps associated with playing a musical instrument, and for muscle control. I once played piano in a concert and, an hour before I was due to go on, while practising, I kept getting cramp in my left hand at a specifically complicated stretch of music. In panic I took two Mag. Phos.

tablets every 10 minutes while I waited to go on and, as a result, I played with not a sign of a cramp! And, coincidentally, I also lost all my pre-concert nerves and tension. Ever since then, before any performance or public speaking event. I take two Mag. Phos. tablets every 10 minutes for about ½ an hour and, as a result I am never nervous or tense. So I add Mag. Phos. for public performances to my list!

- Mag. Phos. is important for arthritis and rheumatism, particularly if the pains are sharp and stabbing. Take it also for chronic conditions of disability and after a fall or concussion.
- I have found this tissue salt a great help for dizzy spells, for the inability to concentrate and for forgetfulness.
- Mag. Phos. seems to have the ability to quench a thirst for sweet cold drinks.
- It somehow gives liveliness to those who tend to sit motionless in stony silence – haven't we all known someone like that? Perhaps Mag. Phos. will lift their spirits, when it is taken in conjunction with Kali. Phos.
- For someone restlessly pacing to and fro, or maybe stammering or having a spell of emotional weepiness, if the throat is so sore you cannot swallow or speak properly – Mag. Phos. taken every 10 minutes will immediately help.
- For a stiff neck, take Mag. Phos. with Kali. Phos. every 20 minutes until the condition eases.

Secondary and complementary salts

Mag. Phos. combines well with Kali. Phos., especially for stress and nervous exhaustion. Mag. Phos. and Silica go well together in helping the body to absorb calcium, and, the duo of Mag. Phos. and Calc. Phos. work wonderfully for pain, spasm and muscular tension.

Herbs that contain Mag. Phos.

- Melissa: an effective antibacterial, it is also a calming antispasmodic, an antidepressant and it also relaxes peripheral blood vessels. It is an effective restorative to the nervous system.

- The mints – peppermint especially: all are antispasmodic and analgesic. Mint promotes bile flow, inhibits vomiting and creates digestive and internal cooling.
- Chamomile: another antispasmodic and anti-inflammatory, this herb is a sedative that calms, unwinds and relaxes mind and body.
- Oats: a restorative nerve tonic and an antidepressant, this cereal imparts a calming quality. Oatstraw makes a relaxing tea and is an excellent bone builder.
- Sage: this must be the real medicinal sage, *Salvia officinalis* – do not use any of the other varieties. Also antispasmodic, it reduces blood sugar levels, acts as a sedative while clearing heat from the body. It also relaxes peripheral blood vessels and has antiseptic properties.
- Nettle: stinging nettle is rich in magnesium and is a circulatory stimulant, a tonic, a diuretic and it also lowers blood sugar levels.
- Dill: this is a good antispasmodic, especially for flatulent colic, griping spasms and for calming indigestion. It also soothes nausea, menstrual pains and helps to stop a baby crying. An old-fashioned – but to my mind – still the best ingredient in gripe water. Incidentally, gripe water isn't just for babies!
- Valerian – in homeopathic form only – is a useful antispasmodic that eases asthma, colic and severe pains in the neck, back and shoulders. It works too on irritable bowel syndrome, menstrual pains and when stress and anxiety cause high blood pressure. Rich in magnesium, it also encourages sleep.
- Dandelion: one of the most mineral-rich herbs known to mankind, it is a superb liver cleanser, a diuretic, an anti-rheumatic and an aid to digestion. Two leaves of dandelion should be eaten daily. Rich in vitamins A, B, C and D, its detoxifying action will clear the body of painful spasm build-up.

Foods rich in Mag. Phos.

Include as many from the following list of foods as possible in your daily diet, if you have any Mag. Phos. deficiency ailments: peas, lettuce, green leafy vegetables, apples, plums, bananas, oranges, grapefruit, naartjies, lemons, almonds, walnuts, lentils, dried and fresh figs, dried beans.

ℳ(agnesium Salad

Try to have this salad three times a week.

1 cup dandelion leaves, chopped
1 cup peas, cooked
1 butter lettuce, torn into small pieces
1 cup green cabbage leaves, thinly shredded
1 cup spinach leaves, thinly shredded
1 cup mustard leaves, thinly shredded, or sprouts
2 cups butter beans, cooked and cooled
juice of 1 lemon
black pepper
a dash of olive oil

Mix everything together and serve immediately. Serves 4

𝒯he constitutional salt

Mag. Phos. is the tissue salt most needed by people born under the astrological sign of Leo. They are usually strong personalities who tend to fearlessly go out and meet the world head on, and they are prone to excess. As a result, tension and stress are part of their daily pattern so Mag. Phos., taken daily and especially at night, will help Leos to cope. It will also help them to relax and feel less pressurised. The B vitamins will also help, especially vitamin B6 – all the Bs work particularly well with Mag. Phos. A combination of Mag. Phos. and vitamin B6 can be bought as a separate tablet at most pharmacies.

$\mathcal{N}$at. Mur.
Natrium Muriaticum
Sodium Muriaticum • Chloride of Soda •
Sodium Chloride (table salt)

Sodium chloride is a constituent of every part of the body. Its main function is as a distributor of water and its role in maintaining the body's water balance is actually by osmosis – the delicate function that shifts moisture in and out of the cells. This powerful affinity to water enables it to control the ebb and flow of body's fluids to maintain a perfect balance. Without Nat. Mur., normal growth and body function cannot take place and, when there is a deficiency of this tissue salt; there is either excessive moisture or excessive dryness.

But, strangely enough, any imbalance cannot be corrected simply by adding extra table salt to one's food. This is because cells cannot utilise the particles of salt unless they are in the accessible attenuated form. It is also important to know that people on a salt-free diet can take Nat. Mur. with complete safety. Approximately two thirds of the body is made of water, so it is easy to understand the vital role Nat. Mur. plays in being the body's water distributor.

Ailments treated
The head
Nat. Mur. is one of the basic headache remedies and, if you have the first hint of a headache, two Nat. Mur. tablets taken every 10 minutes for about 40 minutes, usually clears it completely. A classic and well-documented case occurred in 1955. Sir John Weir, Queen Elizabeth's physician and one of England's greatest homeopathic doctors, publicly stated that, as a medical student, he had suffered

65

from appalling headaches affecting even the sight in one eye. He tried everything to cure himself under the supervision of his teaching doctors. Finally he turned to Dr. Schuessler's salts and immediately his condition started to improve. Within two months of taking Nat. Mur. (on a three times a day basis), he was cured.

At the medical congress at that time, he stated he'd not had a headache for 40 years, thanks to Nat. Mur. As a result of this revelation, doctors started treating patients with Nat. Mur. and found to their astonishment that all sorts of other ailments cleared as well. One headache sufferer found that a lush crop of hair regrew over his bald spot since he had started taking Nat. Mur. consistently for his headaches!

Nat. Mur. is the most important treatment for sunstroke and for the headache caused by being overheated. Dehydration, caused by being overheated, is quickly corrected by two tablets of Nat. Mur., taken every 10-15 minutes, until the headache recedes and energy returns. The same dose is indicated if you wake with a headache every morning.

The eyes and nose

For cataracts, itchy dry eyes, or free-flowing watery fluids (as in hay fever and tears), and itchy eyelids, all these symptoms indicate Nat. Mur. is needed. Other indications include puffiness around and bags under the eyes. For watery, clear nasal catarrh and the start of a cold with sneezing and a copiously runny nose and phlegm in the throat, Nat. Mur. is immediately soothing. Then, at the other extreme, are symptoms of a dry nose, dry, scratchy, painful eyes and a sore throat that also need Nat. Mur. Take two tablets every 10 minutes until the condition clears – usually about an hour. When the eyes are smarting or weak and there is double vision with a headache or the wind causes them to water, Nat. Mur. taken as above will quickly help.

The mouth

A very clear indication of Nat. Mur. deficiency is a mapped tongue and ulcers on the gums. Often Calc. Fluor. is also needed as a secondary salt. If there is excessive salivation – think about teething infants – or extreme dryness in the mouth Nat. Mur. will help. Use also in instances of dribbling or cracks at the corners of the mouth or when fever blisters break out on the lips or around the mouth and nose. A fever blister is surely one of the most painful and irritating of all afflictions that always tends to arrive with its warning sign of a burning sore swelling at the worst possible time. It would happen to me whenever I had to do a television show or give a big public lecture. I learnt to control the problem by taking *elder flower and peppermint tea* (¼ cup fresh elder flowers or ¼ cup fresh peppermint sprigs to 1 cup boiling water. Leave to stand five minutes, strain and sip slowly) three or four times a week. The elder flowers can be dried in summer and stored for use in winter. I would take a cup of the tea every day, alternating elder flowers or peppermint, and I kept it up for a couple of months. At the same time I took two tablets of Nat. Mur. three times a day. Once I had the condition under control I only occasionally take the herb teas, but I often take Nat. Mur. and I have not had a fever blister for years. This is a magical formula. It works – so be persistent.

Digestive system
Those people who take excessive amounts of salt and have a constant craving for it, badly need Nat. Mur. That vast quantity of sodium chloride that has been sprinkled on their food has clogged the cells – it is too coarse to be absorbed and, by the way, may raise the blood pressure. For excessive thirst, or craving for salty foods – we're back to mentioning that 'Coke and chips syndrome' involving too much Coke, too many chips. It's such an easy pick-me-up, but causes serious Nat. Mur. deficiency. So beware! Puffiness around the eyes, swollen, aching finger joints or a post-nasal drip are the reward for that indulgence.

Nat. Mur. plays an important role in the digestive process. Tiny particles of sodium chloride are split up in the peptic glands and, in the process of metabolism, the sodium unites with carbonic acid and enters the blood as sodium carbonate. The chlorine (that by now has dissolved) becomes hydrochloric acid that is present in the stomach and helps to dissolve and process the food we eat. Where there is insufficient hydrochloric acid, there will be indigestion, heartburn and colic. Nat. Mur., taken every five to 10 minutes can quickly correct this – but table salt will make it worse!

In cases of dry, painful constipation and cracks around the anus, or the other extreme, watery diarrhoea, both will respond to two tablets of Nat. Mur. taken every 10-20 minutes for an hour or so, and then every hour until the condition clears. The same treatment can be taken for indigestion and heartburn, and for that bloated feeling or nausea and vertigo. Also remember, Nat. Mur. with Kali. Sulph. helps to regain loss of sense of taste and smell.

The skin

Nat. Mur. is essential in the treatment of eczema, both dry and scaly, itching and weeping, for psoriasis and any ailment that causes blisters and watery discharge on the skin. I have found that a *spritz-spray or lotion* dabbed directly on the area helps immediately, even on babies. Mix 20 drops of Nat. Mur. in ½ cup of water, shake well, then spray or dab onto the area frequently.

Nat. Mur. lotion saved my children from scratching their chicken pox blisters and, when taken six to 10 times a day, the blisters quickly cleared. For chronic facial and scalp eczema, watery pimples, allergy rash, and for a burning feeling on the skin, Nat. Mur. with Calc. Sulph. is particularly effective. For excessive dryness of the scalp, scaly crusts, hives, eruptions on the scalp, and an incessant itch, take Nat. Mur. It is also good for rashes, insect stings and bites, and for allergy swellings. Nat. Mur. comes to the rescue not only as a lotion, but two tablets taken frequently (every 10 minutes for about an hour) will quickly soothe the problem and this dosage can be used for fungus of the nails as well.

For psoriasis that cracks, weeps and itches, make a *cream* by adding 20 drops of liquid Nat. Mur. to ½ cup good aqueous cream, mix well and apply thinly to the area twice a day. You can also make a *lotion* and spray the area often. Take two tablets of Nat. Mur. three to five times a day and this will give tremendous relief. In this way, sodium chloride in its 'triturated' form will give a far more lasting relief than say a swim in the Dead Sea, which for a long time was supposed to help psoriasis sufferers.

To treat shingles – extremely painful and so debilitating – Nat. Mur. together with Mag. Phos., alternating 10 times a day, in conjunction with the lotion sprayed over the area is one of the few things that really helps to ease the pain. The juice of the remarkable herb, Bulbinella (*Bulbine frutescens*) squeezed onto the rash area is also a treatment that brings relief and takes away the pain and burn. Here's a comforting formula for shingles that has proved to be effective: take Nat. Mur., Kali. Mur. and Kali. Phos – two tablets of each three times a day – and twice a day, two tablets each of Calc. Phos. and Ferrum Phos. Take this combination daily for at least three weeks, even when the symptoms ease. Usually perfect health is restored in four weeks' time.

For oily patches on the face and for thin white scaly patches and for facial skin that is both oily and excessively dry, Nat. Mur. is needed both in lotion form and tablets taken three times a day.

Circulatory system

For cold extremities, blue hands and feet, and a great sensitivity to cold and a dislike of being either too cold or too hot, Nat. Mur. is needed. Use it also for treating haemorrhoids using a lotion or cream, made as described above, together with two tablets taken four to eight times a day.

Urinary system

For those who have to make frequent trips to the toilet with resulting thin, watery, colourless urine accompanied often by thin, watery, painless diarrhoea, Nat. Mur. is indicated, two tablets four to eight times a day. These symptoms are often accompanied by an insatiable thirst that Nat. Mur. will restore to normal.

Female problems

Nat. Mur. should be considered for irregular menstruation or missed periods, especially if this is the result of over-excitement, stress or unhappiness and excessive tearfulness. Irritability, nervous jerking and twitching during sleep are also often experienced. Connect all the symptoms and often a Nat. Mur. deficiency will emerge. Treat by taking two tablets of Nat. Mur., six times during the day or more

69

if required. For that dip in depression with sadness and anxiety a few days before the period begins, Nat. Mur. will lift the mood, when taken as above. For uterine cramps, take Mag. Phos. with Nat. Mur. and, for burning dryness of the vagina and that heavy, bloated feeling in the lower abdomen and profuse menstruation, all these unpleasant conditions will respond to Nat. Mur.

Many women experience a decreased libido, a diminished desire for sex, and often this is accompanied by a headache, which isn't a joke – it literally happens. It's known as 'Not now, darling, I have a headache' syndrome. Two tablets of Nat. Mur. taken three to six times a day, usually corrects this. And, remember Nat. Mur. is the best headache treatment! And, for the very opposite of decreased libido – nymphomania – a combination of Nat. Mur., Calc. Phos. and Silica – two tablets of each taken up to 10 times a day – to calm the desire. For leucorrhea – a vaginal discharge causing a burning itch and also loss of pubic hair – wash with Nat. Mur. lotion and take Nat. Mur. with Calc. Phos. six times a day.

During pregnancy
Nat. Mur. is a great comfort at this time, not just to help with feeling better, but also for that shaky 'gone' feeling in the stomach. It is also indicated for the temporary abhorrence of certain foods with associated nausea and vomiting. If there's hair loss or haemorrhoids during the pregnancy, slow labour, morning sickness, urine spurt while coughing (combine with Ferrum Phos.), and vomiting of frothy phlegm during morning sickness all respond to Nat. Mur. – two tablets four to 10 times daily.

And later, after birth, if the baby refuses the breast take Nat. Mur. with Silica and if the nipples are cracked and sore – all respond to Nat. Mur. taken up to 10 times during the day.

How you feel
Through the years I have made pages of notes on the precious tissue salts and my notes on Nat. Mur., verified by my Swiss doctor many years ago, are copious. I made a long list of the extraordinary ability of Nat. Mur. to lift and lighten moods. If you have, or recognise in someone else, any of the following symptoms or conditions, Nat.

Mur. should be your daily companion:
- irritability and quickness to anger, a 'short fuse' and road rage!
- moods when you feel gloomy, taciturn, depressed, dull, distracted, indifferent, joyless, impatient, rushed and aggressive
- a feeling of despair with hopelessness about the future
- awkwardness, make mistakes easily, anxious with a fluttering heart
- a brooding or low-spirited nature, or an attitude that is hateful, mean, conniving and vindictive.

We all know people who have bad moods, as described above, and we may well recognise some of the mean and angry symptoms in ourselves from time to time. Two tablets of Nat. Mur. taken six times a day will do much to restore a more pleasant outlook and nature. Don't ignore this important tissue salt. Whether the uncontrollable bad moods are regularly experienced by you or by someone close to you – our world would be a better place if we all took Nat. Mur. on a daily basis. Do something about it.

General symptoms
Any of the following ailments indicate a deficiency of Nat. Mur. in the body: allergic rhinitis, hay fever, an endocrine imbalance, insomnia, asthma, jerking limbs during sleep, diabetes, sinusitis, stinging piles, chronic syphilis or chronic gonorrhoea, irregular heart beat, hysterical spasms, debility, swollen ankles, swollen limbs, constipation, alopecia (hair loss), poor immunity, cracking joints, arthritis, warts, postnatal depression, clinical depression, grief, tearfulness, sleeping sickness, gastro-enteritis, sneezing constantly, thirst and sweating, hot, stuffy, itchy ears caused by an allergic reaction, and frequent over-indulgence in alcohol.

Secondary and complementary salts
The main tissue salt that works well in conjunction with Nat. Mur. is Ferrum Phos., but Nat. Phos. and Kali. Phos. also work well as does Silica. Calc. Phos. also combines well with Nat. Mur. and is an excellent 'tonic' salt few of us can do without.

Herbs that contain Nat. Mur.

- Comfrey: an old-fashioned healer, comfrey is rich in Nat. Mur. and is particularly good as a *skin lotion*. Pour one cup of boiling water over ¼ cup of fresh chopped comfrey leaves. Leave to stand for five minutes, then strain and use as a spray-on treatment or dab onto the affected area.
- Mustard, calendula, chickweed, celery, thyme, origanum and marjoram: all are rich in Nat. Mur. and can be used in the diet as a natural flavour to replace salt. To make your own *salt-free seasoning*, combine ½ cup each dried thyme, celery leaves, origanum and marjoram leaves and mustard leaves. Add ½ cup each of sesame seeds and mustard seeds. Mix everything together. Every time you need extra flavour in a dish, take a little of the mixture and pound in a pestle and mortar.
- Garden violets, valerian (use in homeopathic form only), melissa and chamomile: all these herbs contain Nat. Mur. and are natural tranquillisers. They will also help to stop sneezing, headaches, sinusitis and relieve insomnia. To make a *tea* pour a cup of boiling water over a ¼ cup fresh leaves and flowers of any of these herbs. Leave to stand for five minutes, then strain. Take one to two cups daily.

Foods rich in Nat. Mur.

- Seafood – be careful as some people develop an intolerance or an allergy to certain types of seafood. Also be aware of monosodium glutamate, used in salty flavourings and in a lot of Chinese dishes. This is the cause of many allergic reactions that start with hay fever and wheezing and can lead to serious allergic reaction like seafood allergy. Include fish in the diet twice a week.
- Cabbage, spinach, parsley, asparagus, carrots, lentils, beetroot and meat – especially beef and mutton – are rich in Nat. Mur. Almonds, sesame seeds, figs, apples, strawberries and buckwheat all are rich in Nat. Mur. and some should be included in the daily diet.

Nat. Mur. Health Drink

This is the most vital health drink I know and is superb for convalescents and anyone trying to boost their immune system. I try to take it three times a week in winter to fight colds and 'flu. The vegetables are best grown organically and, if this drink is taken every day with Nat. Mur., that weary fatigue and tired-when-you-wake-up feeling – that no pep pills can correct – will become a thing of the past! Someone who is abundantly supplied with Nat. Mur. will show no signs of excessive thirst or any of the above symptoms.

In a juice extractor, press through:

2 carrots, cleaned and peeled

2 apples, peeled

1 raw beetroot, peeled

3 beetroot leaves

3 sticks of celery

4 sprigs parsley

Catch the juice in a glass and drink it immediately. Serves 1.

Building the soil

Many years ago there was a marvellous natural soil additive used by farmers on an annual basis to spread over their productive land. Known as 'stone meal', it was composed of finely crushed rock containing all the mineral elements (including Nat. Mur.) necessary for a chemically balanced soil. And, as such, it was capable of producing natural, chemically perfect food, which in turn contributed to perfect health. When sprinkled as a mulch on to the soil, the stone meal also acted as an insect deterrent for when the mineral content of the soil is in perfect balance, plants grow strongly and there is nothing to support insect life, which thrives on decay and decomposition.

It helps to maintain the soil moisture, so gardens spread with stone meal flourish, it absorbs the dew and the rain, and so in times of drought crops can still be maintained. Isn't it time we looked at nature's minerals and reintroduce the natural soil builders to nourish us all?

The constitutional salt

This is the tissue salt most needed by the astrological sign of Aquarius, the water carrier. Nat. Mur. must be taken daily, as so many of the above symptoms are particularly evident in the personality and health of people born under this sign.

Often an Aquarian shows signs of impatience, even as a young child. My old Swiss doctor called Nat. Mur. the 'impatience salt' or the 'aggression salt'. So, for every Aquarian and all of us besides, in order to make life more peaceful around us remember to take Nat. Mur.!

I frequently deal with very difficult people who impatiently reel off their symptoms, and a Nat. Mur. deficiency is always predominant. With humour I make them read my Grandmother's poem, which she made us read when we were impatient, and I suggest a good few doses of Nat. Mur.:

Guard my tongue oh Lord this day

Let my words spread peace I pray,

Conflict can so often start

If spoken from a hasty heart

This unruly tongue please curb,

Lest I disrupt or I disturb.

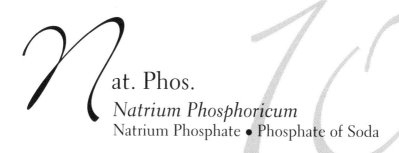

at. Phos.
Natrium Phosphoricum
Natrium Phosphate • Phosphate of Soda

Nat. Phos. is characterised by the following functions: it is the biochemical antacid, acid neutraliser and acid/alkaline balancer. The main action of Nat. Phos. in the body is to break down lactic acid that, if not decomposed or catalysed, will irritate the tissues to the extent of pain. So, in breaking up lactic acid into carbonic acid and water, Nat. Phos. serves to keep the carbonic acid in the blood until it reaches the lungs. It is then exhaled in the breath, thus releasing it and reducing acid in the whole body. The action of Nat. Phos. also prevents the viscosity of bile in the gall bladder and the gall duct. It assists the assimilation of fats and prevents a bilious feeling or worse, jaundice, due to an insufficient amount of bile.

Uric acid is present in the blood and Nat. Phos. keeps it soluble. But, without Nat. Phos., uric acid combines with any carbonic acid that may be present, resulting in an extremely over-acid condition where acid gets deposited in the joints, which then become painfully inflamed.

Nat. Phos. is present in the blood, the muscles, the nerves, the brain cells as well as in the all the body fluids. So, it is easy to understand how Nat. Phos. plays such a role in digestion. It is the major remedy and it combines well with the other 'Natrium' salts and particularly Nat. Sulph. to keep the digestive system healthy.

Ailments treated

Digestive system

Digestion is vital to health. If food is not digested properly the body cannot utilise it nor eliminate properly. Symptoms that indicate Nat. Phos. is in limited supply include a feeling of heat or churning in the stomach, a dislike of otherwise favourite foods, raiding the refrigerator at night, not feeling satisfied after a meal, and being picky or peckish constantly. And, then there's that painful sour reflux, stomach ulcers, dyspepsia, repeated heartburn attacks, nausea, belching of sour gases, vomiting up of sour foods, discomfort and that bloated feeling, especially after eating citrus, and perhaps there's also a yellowish coating at the back of the tongue.

If stools burn or there is sour smelling diarrhoea and even worms, are all indications that Nat. Phos. is badly deficient. Replenish by taking two tablets as soon as symptoms occur, followed by two more and then take two every 10 minutes for about 40 minutes, or until the discomfort disappears. Usually symptoms ease quickly.

If indigestion is your problem, keep a bottle of Nat. Phos. in your pocket or bag to take *prior* to a meal. Suck two tablets *after* the meal just as you would take any commercial antacid. The great difference is that Nat. Phos. clears acid build-up from the whole body, not just the stomach, therefore correcting it in the long term.

Where children are eating wrongly or over-indulging in sweet things – such as artificially coloured and flavoured, over-sugared junk food that is generally served at children's parties – give 10 drops of Nat. Phos. to ½ cup of warm water, or dissolve four tablets in the water and let the child sip it slowly before the party, if possible, and again the same dose after the party. Give another dose before bedtime. Acid build-up, caused by consuming all that rubbish, will not only be cleared but you will not have an overwrought hyperactive little monster!

But please don't imagine you can eat junk food with impunity and resolve the problem by taking Nat. Phos.! Diet is very important, this is something I learnt early on. I brought up my three children on a farm a good distance from any town. As they started to grow I felt they needed to come in contact with other children of their own age and so they were invited to my friends' children's parties. But, with only good, wholesome food on their table at home, their eyes were as big as saucers at the gaudy array of party food that everyone was tucking into. After a while I noticed they were behaving as badly as the rest of the little hooligans, tearing about and screaming and fighting each other. By the time we set off for home, my normally happy youngsters had become a bunch of monsters fighting, crying and being impossible.

After another party visit finished with the same performance, I quickly dosed them with Nat. Phos. as they fought their way into the car to go home. I then became clever and dosed them before the next party, during it, and, as we set off for home. I also added a dose of Nat. Mur. and Kali. Phos. on the trip home to help the bad moods, and this way, I managed to turn them back into the happy little farm children they'd always been. Those three tissue salts accompanied us everywhere and when anyone behaved badly, the others would rush to find the salts and dose the offender!

The skeleton

Nat. Phos. will help conditions such as rheumatic and arthritic joint pains, chronic and acute inflammatory arthritis, creaking and cracking joints, stiffness, a weakness in the legs, chronic backache and acute gout – the common factor is acidity. Two tablets of Nat. Phos., taken every 15-20 minutes until the immediate discomfort goes – about an hour – and thereafter four to eight times a day, will give comforting relief. Take Nat. Phos. combined with Nat. Sulph. – they work together well – and you'll find wonderful relief. For an acute attack of gout, take two tablets of Ferrum Phos. as well. A cup of *stinging nettle tea* will also help. Add ¼ cup fresh leaves to one cup boiling water. Allow the tea to stand for five minutes, then strain and sip slowly. Take three cups per day in the acute stage over three days, then one cup a day for the following week.

The head

For a headache that is accompanied by sour belching and heartburn, or vomiting and gastric problems – diarrhoea and colic – take Nat. Phos. and Nat. Sulph. together to restore the normal processes. Take two tablets of each under the tongue every 10 minutes until the pain subsides (usually within about 30 minutes).

The eyes

Nat. Phos. is excellent for treating conjunctivitis and a cream-coloured discharge that forms a crust around the rim of the eye.

77

Dr. Schuessler's case histories proved any inflammatory condition around or in the eyes could be quickly soothed by taking two tablets of Nat. Phos. every 15 minutes for about an hour, and thereafter every hour until it clears.

To make a *lotion* to cool red eyelids, mix 10 drops of Nat. Phos. in ½ cup warm water and dab it onto the eyelids frequently – note *not* into the eyes – until the inflammation clears.

The skin

Nat. Phos. fights excess acidity, which aggravates or causes rose rash, hives, itchiness, eczema, yellowing skin and a dry, scaly scalp. The formulas of many modern shampoos create an acid/alkaline balance so the scalp becomes neutral and the hair more manageable. Nat. Phos. works on the acid balance to improve the appearance of the hair by reducing the internal acidity.

For itchy hands, itchy anus or itchy shins, Nat. Phos. is excellent and can be made into a *lotion* to dab onto the affected area. Add 20 drops of liquid Nat. Phos. to ½ cup of warm water, mix well and apply frequently.

The teeth

This may come as a surprise! Anyone, child or adult, who sleeps restlessly and grinds their teeth in their sleep, is in need of Nat. Phos. (To substantiate this need, there will be other bodily ailments, for example an itchy anus, that will also indicate over-acidity and the need for Nat. Phos.) Two tablets three or four times a day and particularly at night, will help.

Female problems

Cystitis and vaginal secretions that are acid and create irritation, or have an unpleasantly sour smell, indicate the need for Nat. Phos. The same applies to redness accompanied by an itch. Two tablets taken three or four times a day usually clears the condition, but if you suffer from one or all of the above complaints, make a lotion and use it to wash and douche with. There is instant relief with a *lotion* mixed with 50 drops liquid Nat. Phos. in one litre of warm water, to which ½ a cup of apple cider vinegar is added. Mix well and use as a dab-on lotion and/or a douche. Repeat the treatment with a fresh lotion mixture over the next two days, but keep taking the tablets for at least a month.

General symptoms

If a feeling of dizziness, nausea or vertigo is experienced, or perhaps being unable to lift your head for fear of falling, or not being able to stand up straight, all these unpleasant symptoms could be due to a lack of Nat. Phos. Take two tablets every 15 minutes initially, for an hour to ease the condition. Then, take two tablets every half-hour for the following three hours and two tablets every two hours taken thereafter should bring relief.

Nat. Phos. is essential to treat yellow jaundice and it needs to be taken seriously as this tissue salt helps to cleanse the liver. Start off with two tablets every 15 minutes for two hours then follow up with two tablets every two hours until the pain and lassitude subside.

Sexual excesses and vices need to be controlled and normalised with Nat. Phos. Dr. James Kent advised two tablets to be taken four to six times a day. He also reportedly found Nat. Phos. excellent for patients in a fret from mental exertion or mental fuzziness.

I use and recommend this tissue salt for exam-time worries, tension and fear, and every student responds well. This salt is also helpful for people who sometimes become angry over trivial matters or are easily angered – the short-fuse syndrome – or perhaps are over-anxious at night with night sweats and worries or become unsociable.

I always know when I'm short on Nat. Phos. I wake at 3 a.m. in a sweat of anxiety with a pounding heart following a vivid nightmare. This feeling is accompanied with my fourth and little fingers on both hands feeling stiff and sore and my shoulders and neck aching. If you recognise these symptoms, I have a *magic formula*: I reach for the phosphates among the tissue salts, these being salts no. 2, 4, 6, 8 and especially no. 10. I take two tablets of each of the first four and three of no. 10. I dissolve them in ½ a glass of warm water and sip it slowly, holding every mouthful for a few moments in my mouth before swallowing. I then turn over and go to back to sleep

79

and somehow I awake refreshed. Throughout the next day, every couple of hours, I take two tablets of Nat. Phos. And, during that night I have no nightmares.

Ailments affecting the urinary system need Nat. Phos. For instance, gallstones, kidney pain and acid urine, nephritis, kidney and bladder weakness, all can be alleviated with this important tissue salt. It also helps calm a general bilious feeling, a skin that is blotchy or a face flushed after eating. An inflamed or ulcerated throat will also respond favourably to this tissue salt, as does an acid, itchy, cream-coloured nasal discharge. And, if you suffer from halitosis and/or body odour Nat. Phos. will also help this unsociable condition.

The conditions that this salt helps are diverse and range from inflamed conditions, such as fibrositis and sciatica, to allergic eczema and morning sickness. And don't forget that horrid 'liverish' feeling – remember Nat. Phos. is a liver cleanser – all these conditions should all respond well to taking two tablets of Nat. Phos. three or four times a day.

If an uncontrolled spurt of urine is experienced when sneezing or coughing, Nat. Phos. helps to curb it. Combine two tablets each of Calc. Phos., Kali. Phos., Nat. Mur. and Nat. Phos., taken four times a day. Suck slowly and this treatment should be kept up for 20 months to help strengthen the bladder.

For smokers intent on kicking the cigarette habit, Nat. Phos. and Nat. Sulph. will be of great benefit. Take two tablets of each six times a day. And, for osteo-arthritis the same dose will ease that constant pain.

It is recorded that certain doctors involved in the treatment of morphine addicts noted that Nat. Phos. was a great help. For two months the addict received a daily injection of Nat. Phos. just under the skin. Then, as the need for morphine lessened, Nat. Phos. was increased. Within three months the patient was cured. This occured many years ago and, at the time, it impressed me greatly, thus reaffirming my belief in these amazing salts.

Here is just a small but important aspect to consider. I lecture to several beauty schools and always teach the students that Nat. Phos., used as a *lotion* in combination with Calc. Phos. and Kali.

80

Sulph., will help to produce new skin cells. Twenty drops of each in a cup of warm water, applied with a spray (spritz) bottle to the face after washing, will act as a beauty tonic. At the same time, two tablets should be taken, twice a day every day to encourage new skin regeneration. This is a superb beauty treatment.

Secondary and complementary salts

Nat. Phos. and Nat. Sulph. are excellent partners. Nat. Phos. is such a superb digestive that it will enhance the assimilation of any other tissue salt. If the other cell salts are not immediately showing results, they are likely to act faster with added Nat. Phos.

Mag. Phos. and Calc. Phos. together help Nat. Phos. maintain a good acid-alkaline balance, so they should be included in the occasional treatment as well.

Herbs that contain Nat. Phos.

Coriander, caraway, cumin, anise, ginger – all these herbs are excellent aids to the digestion. Chew a few seeds or make a *tea*. Add 1 teaspoon of seeds or three or four thin slices of ginger in 1 cup boiling water. Stand, stir well, then strain and sip slowly.

Lucerne, fennel, any of the mints, violets, dill, basil, nettles and lemon balm are all digestive aids and they detoxify the system. These herbs work like a tonic on the whole system, cleansing, releasing spasm and flushing the kidneys and bladder. Eat fresh parsley daily. To make a *herb tea* of any of the above herbs: add ¼ cup leaves to one cup boiling water, stand for five minutes, then strain and sip slowly. Take two to three cups of any of these specific herbs every day in acute conditions, but I vary these and drink a few different herb teas daily.

Foods rich in Nat. Phos.

Rice, celery, beetroot, apples, peaches, apricots, pawpaw, quinces, mealies, raspberries, mulberries, plain yoghurt, strawberries, raisins and grapes, carrots and asparagus. In-season watermelon helps to

81

flush acidity, and remember that, difficult though it may be to understand, lemons are not acidic within the body but they become alkaline, as does apple cider vinegar. Both these fluids are very beneficial in maintaining the acid-alkaline balance of the body. Two teaspoons of apple cider vinegar (use fresh – not in capsule form) in 1 glass of water taken daily – not necessarily first thing in the morning – will greatly ease acidity. A refreshing glass of iced water with 2 teaspoons of apple cider vinegar at the end of an exhaustingly hot day is a wonderful reviver!

 The constitutional salt

This is the salt most needed by people born under the astrological sign of Libra. When Librans are anxious or worried, they are engulfed by indecision – those emotions build up acidity and the acidity causes all the problems listed above. Librans also need to attend to their diet. Incorrect eating for them will cause much discomfort. Non-acid forming foods are essential to maintain their equilibrium. We all become acidic if we eat incorrectly, or worry, with anger and fear, and all these conditions require Nat. Phos. But this is particularly a Libran weakness, so no Libran should ever go a day without taking Nat. Phos.

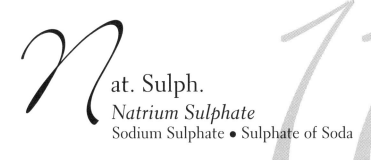

$\mathcal{N}$at. Sulph.
Natrium Sulphate
Sodium Sulphate • Sulphate of Soda

Nat. Sulph. is characterised by the following functions: a cell cleanser, particularly to detoxify the liver and as a decongestant. This tissue salt has the extraordinary ability to act as a regulator, in that it controls the density of intercellular fluids by eliminating excess water and removing toxins from body fluids. Nat. Sulph. provides the greatest help to the liver by ensuring there is an adequate supply of healthy bile that flows unimpeded. It is therefore vitally important that the body has an adequate supply of this tissue salt.

Sodium sulphate is produced by the action of sulphuric acid on ordinary table salt. What is particularly interesting in this regard, is that this process occurs naturally in vast quantities in many of Russia's salt lakes. When it is chemically manufactured, it is known as Glauber's salt but, as a cell salt remedy, it is obtained from its natural source.

Just as sodium chloride attracts water to the body's tissues, sodium sulphate clears it away in its role as the waste remover and cleanser of the cells. Ailments that are aggravated by moisture, such as humidity, damp weather, seaside mist, moist earth – all will improve by taking this tissue salt. It also has a stimulating effect on the cell linings, as well as on the nerves and the structure of the bile ducts. Nat. Sulph. is also advantageous to the pancreas and intestines, as well as to the filtering tubes of the whole urinary system, where it clears toxins, flushing them out as waste-carrying urine.

In its role of secreting and stimulating fluids through the pancreas, Nat. Sulph. is of considerable importance to diabetics. It should be considered, with the doctor's approval, as a long-term aid in assisting the action of the pancreas. Note: Diabetics need to take biochemic tissue salts in liquid form as the tablets are in a milk lactose base.

Ailments treated

Body symptoms

An interesting observation for those in need of Nat. Sulph, a long-standing need, is the build-up of non-budging obesity especially of the thighs, the abdomen and the buttocks, the typical cellulite look of dimples and bulges that cause most women to despair. As these areas are so prone to weight build-up – it's always the first sign – the tissues become overloaded with fats and fluids that tenaciously lodge there, creating the dreaded cellulite.

The head

In the case of a debilitating nauseous headache, vomiting, sour gastric belching and a queasy stomach – almost like a migraine – Nat. Sulph. combined with Nat. Phos. is extremely comforting. Take two tablets of each every seven to 10 minutes until the condition eases. Nat. Sulph. is also indicated if your eyes focus sluggishly in combination with a headache, or when there is a thick, yellow discharge at the corners of the eyes.

My Swiss doctor friend also advised that Nat. Sulph. be taken for any head injury that causes congestion and that blocked-up, fuzzy feeling. It is also good for head wounds that suppurate and are slow to heal. Take two tablets four to six times a day. Dr. Schuessler recommended Nat. Sulph. also for the inability to concentrate or think clearly – remember its waste-removing ability.

Respiratory system

Up until my late-thirties I was a bad asthmatic. Many herbal remedies helped, but I still relied on those heart-racing bronchodilators until I seriously looked at homeopathic respiratory treatments. As a result, I went onto a sustained tissue salt support treatment and appreciate Nat. Sulph. as a great friend – a natural asthmatic treatment – especially for those damp days when my chest was tight. Nat. Sulph., taken during the day up to 15 times, helped enormously.

For that tight wheezy cough and thick phlegm and coughing up yellow sputum, Nat. Sulph. comes to the rescue. If you suffer from coughing fits, dissolve six tablets of Nat. Sulph. in ½ cup of warm water and sip it frequently. If you consider the fact that Nat. Sulph. is able to remove twice its bulk in water-containing waste products and then flush it out, it's no wonder long-standing asthma cases such as mine can usually be helped. Nat. Sulph. has the ability to heal the mucous membranes, and that thick nasal discharge can quickly be cleared.

$\mathcal{L}$et's talk about 'flu

Dr. Charles Vaught, a chest specialist, found he could successfully ease the symptoms of 'flu – in its earliest stages – by taking massive doses of Nat. Sulph. at the first signs of sneezing, a runny nose, tight cough, aches and pains, etc. The formula he found worked best was the combination of Calc. Fluor. (tissue salt no. l), Ferrum Phos. (no. 4), Kali. Mur. (no. 5), Nat. Mur. (no. 9) and Nat. Sulph. (no. 11). So that combination – 1, 4, 5, 9, 11 – has remained in my head, as each one of these salts has a particular role to play and Dr. Vaught found no. 11 to be his particular favourite. His advised remedy was to take one to two tablets of each every 15 minutes for the first two hours, thereafter every ½ an hour for the next three hours, and every hour following until the symptoms subsided. Alternatively, mix 10 tablets of each and dissolve together in ½ cup of warm water and sip frequently.

Digestive system

Nat. Sulph. can play an effective role in treating a whole variety of digestive problems, and particularly problems with the gall bladder and also the liver. If you have, or you observe anyone else with a blue-red nose, this is a symptom indicating there is a problem with the liver and not, as you might have thought, an over-indulgence in alcohol. (Although Nat. Sulph. is also helpful the next morning in treating a hangover!)

Throughout the world sugar consumption has increased so drastically that our bodies now show symptoms of overload. Diabetes is common, both in adults and young children, and some dieticians are convinced it is due to increased sugar intake. Think of the sweets and cakes on offer at every corner café and supermarket, and now even at petrol stations across the country. How do we stop our children from being sugar addicts when there is so much on offer? Diabetes responds well to Nat. Sulph. – 10 drops in ½ a glass of water, taken three times a day. And, foods containing Nat. Sulph. are hugely important in the everyday diet. If you have a bitter taste in the mouth and the breath smells, or if you are often bilious and vomit green, bitter bile, Nat. Sulph. is in dire need.

Other symptoms include abdominal bloating, and colic, and an intolerance of tight clothing around the abdomen. If you have an intense thirst for cold, sweet drinks and there is much flatulence, especially after consuming the cold drinks, then Nat. Sulph. is required. Another indication is when there is watery diarrhoea, sometimes alternating with bouts of constipation and even a distended liver that is tender to the touch. You'll notice a grey-brown coating to the tongue. All these symptoms indicate the need for Nat. Sulph. – two tablets taken every 20-30 minutes until the condition eases. For best results, take it with Nat. Phos. or Nat. Mur., depending on the symptoms.

The skeleton

The health of the bony structure of the body is very important to our well-being. The lower back, shoulders, knees, ankles, hips, all the joints in fact can seize in rheumatic pains with cracking sounds, especially due to moisture and humidity. All bone-related complaints will subside when two tablets of Nat. Sulph. are taken every 20-30 minutes, or until the pain and stiffness eases. Nat. Sulph. is also a great panacea for jarring falls where the joints take strain. It also helps when you feel cold at night – specially the feet and hands. *Take Nat. Sulph. to keep your extremities warm.* For an old head injury, and particularly after an accident involving an injury to the head, Nat. Sulph. helps and it is also ideal after dental treatment where a painful jaw is experienced.

Female problems

Nat. Sulph. works directly on mucous membranes and one of the most excruciating discomforts is a genital itch that responds to no amount of washing or soothing ointments. Often it is deep-seated and accompanied by a sour-smelling discharge. A *lotion* and *douche* made by dissolving 10 tablets of Nat. Sulph. in ½ a litre of warm water with ½ cup of apple cider vinegar, dab on often, will quickly ease pain, and two tablets taken four to eight times during the day will quickly clear both the itch and the discharge. Also include two helpings equal to about ¾ cup of plain yoghurt daily.

The skin

Does your skin sometimes itch after you've undressed to get into bed or take a bath? Or, perhaps you have a complaint such as a chafed area of skin or itchy, watery secretions or scabies or crusty rashes or eczema. Use Nat. Sulph. as a *lotion* – six to 10 tablets dissolved in two cups of water – applied liberally to the area, dabbed on with cotton-wool pads, or applied directly from a spray bottle. In addition, take two tablets four times a day, to quickly ease the irritation.

How you feel

A deficiency in Nat. Sulph. results in the following emotional symptoms: despondency, fear or dread, nightmares, feelings of discouragement, melancholia, manic depression, the aching feeling of being alone and unloved. It also helps conditions such as mental weakness due to head injury and concussion, dizziness, hopelessness, and a tendency to want to commit suicide, also for that inability to get started in the mornings. Two tablets of Nat. Sulph. taken four to six times a day will relieve all these unhappy symptoms.

For the insomniac, Nat. Sulph. is a non-addictive sleeping potion. If you have anxiety-ridden dreams, nightmares with frequent restless, anxious wakings, or wake in the small hours and are unable to get to sleep again, take two Nat. Sulph. tablets every hour from 5 p.m. until bedtime. Practise this every day until the sleep pattern corrects and sleeplessness is something of the past.

By establishing this regime, other emotions will also correct themselves. Here, I am referring to irritability, short tempers, depression and despair, anxiety and abrupt behaviour – they will all ease and gradually become less frequent. You will feel more confident and refreshed each morning and you will be able to cope better with the fast pace of modern life. You will be able to reject those anxiety-ridden feelings of overload.

Mood-lifter and natural tranquilliser

By taking Nat. Sulph. with Kali. Phos., Calc. Phos. and Nat. Mur., you could find an excellent mood-lifter and natural tranquilliser that makes the greatest difference to how you cope and how you feel.

Other symptoms

There are numerous and diverse conditions where Nat. Sulph. will help. Whether taken alone or in combination with other tissue salts, it provides very beneficial results.

Take it in the treatment of warts on any part of the body and for whitlows. Make a *lotion* by dissolving six tablets in ½ a cup of warm water and apply liberally and frequently to the area.

It also helps in cases of urine retention and incontinence, or a burning sensation in the nose and mouth. The same applies if there is earache with noises in the ears, or a burning feeling in the soles of the feet and also for soft swellings, swollen feet, acute sciatica and backache, and even to subdue vomiting during pregnancy. All these conditions will respond when Nat. Sulph. is taken in conjunction with Nat. Phos. and Kali. Phos.

Take it when there is too much milk during breastfeeding and bilious fevers, and green thick catarrhs, or for yellow skin and freckles and liver spots on the hands and face, also for worm infestation – all need Nat. Sulph., usually two tablets taken four to six times a day.

In *leukaemia*, where the leukocytes remain too long in the blood before disintegrating, Nat. Sulph. withdraws their moisture content and sets the disintegration process in motion. On blood analysis, it was found there was an insufficiency of Nat. Sulph. and, with extra dosages, it could help considerably under a doctor's supervision.

Nat. Sulph. is the one tissue salt that is extremely important for treating *malaria*. During the early stages take two tablets every hour and then as the symptoms ease, take two tablets six to 10 times a day until the patient feels better. Don't treat yourself, but take Nat. Sulph. with other prescribed medication, with the doctor's knowledge.

Nat. Sulph. with Calc. Sulph. and Silica will also sweeten bad breath, and, when taken with Ferrum Phos., it will help to raise very low blood pressure – take two tablets of each three times a day. Take Nat. Sulph. for athlete's foot in conjunction with Kali. Sulph. – these two are an excellent combination, when two tablets of each are taken four to six times a day. At the same time, apply a *lotion* made from six tablets of each dissolved in a cup of warm water. Apply frequently.

Secondary and complementary salts

Nat. Sulph.'s closest companion is Nat. Phos., which complements its action especially in the case of over-acidic or liverish conditions. Similarly, Nat. Sulph. and Nat. Mur. are closely linked both having an important role in regulating the body's water metabolism. And, in combination with Kali Mur, Nat. Sulph. proves vital in the function of organs and glands. Finally, remember the need to lift the spirits and remove congestion and congested thoughts, bad moods and suffering – Kali. Phos. and Calc. Phos. together with Nat. Sulph. will lift the whole personality and spirit.

Herbs that contain Nat. Sulph.

- Burdock (*Arctium lappa*): an amazing herb that is both anti-rheumatic and a diuretic, it has a mild laxative effect and also contains natural antibiotic substances.
- Mullein (*Verbascum thapsus*): a superb expectorant, a wound healer, anti-inflammatory and a light sedative. Flowers and leaves have these qualities and, in Europe, it is one of the primary respiratory treatments, as it removes mucous build-up.
- Yarrow (*Achillea millefolia*): this is an anti-allergenic herb, an antispasmodic and an anti-inflammatory. It is a digestive tonic that stimulates bile flow and the circulation in general. It can also help to lower high blood pressure, is a good diuretic and acts as a blood tonic.
- Parsley: an excellent cleanser, diuretic and tonic herb. Eat 2 tablespoons fresh parsley daily.
- Celery: a general cleanser, it flushes toxins from the kidneys and liver and is an effective diuretic and an anti-rheumatic. It increases

uric acid secretions and is an excellent urinary antiseptic. Eat fresh daily. Make a *tea* of any of these herbs by pouring one cup of boiling water over ½ cup fresh leaves. Leave to stand five minutes and strain. Take two to three cups daily until the infection clears.

- Cayenne pepper: an antibacterial and a circulatory stimulant, it is rich in vitamins A, B1 and C. This vegetable is invaluable for removing a build-up of waste produce. Like mullein, it clears mucous. Use as red pepper or eat fresh on bread.
- Horseradish: – high in vitamin C, it is a good diuretic and stimulates perspiration and digestion while pepping up the circulation. It is a good expectorant and a marvellous natural treatment for both urinary tract and respiratory infections. Use as a sauce or add leaves to soups.

Foods rich in Nat. Sulph.

Include as many of the following foods as you can in the daily diet. The cabbage family – broccoli, Brussels sprouts, kale, cabbage and cauliflower – especially the green outer leaves. I grow a row of winter cabbages that hardly ever reach a head in size, as I am so busy picking off the outer leaves for quick steaming with lemon juice or for stir-fries. Onions and their green succulent leaves, leeks, beetroot and beetroot leaves, pumpkin and pumpkin flowers plus the tips of the pumpkin vines, green peppers, paprika, cucumber, bananas and apples.

 The constitutional tissue salt

This is the salt most needed by those born under the astrological sign of Taurus. Often Tauruaeans have a sluggish metabolism, and it's easy for them to put on weight. Also, Taureans can easily become depressed, and eat too much as compensation. Nat. Sulph. is a most effective metabolism stimulant, clearing so much that is not wanted – waste and congested thoughts. Nat. Sulph. really is a mover and shaker and we should all be aware of the importance of 'cleaning out'.

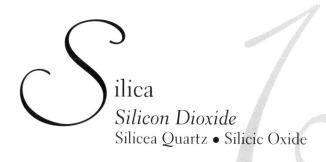

$\mathcal{S}$ ilica
Silicon Dioxide
Silicea Quartz • Silicic Oxide

Silica is a slow-acting yet profound remedy in that its key functions are as a toxin eliminator and cell cleanser – it is known as 'the homeopathic surgeon'.

When the skin is not perspiring sufficiently for toxins to be eliminated, Silica is deficient. This tissue salt should naturally be present in the skin, the hair, nails, bones, blood, bile and in the nerve sheaths and mucous membranes. It is the main constituent of all the connective tissue cells and, as connective tissue covers the brain, the spinal cord and the nerve fibres, an imbalance of Silica causes poor memory, absent-mindedness, slow and difficult thought patterns, as well as pain and swelling and ponderous movements.

In the early years of my work with tissue salts, I remember the most important words about a specific tissue salt I wrote in huge red letters – and for Silica I wrote, 'Silica gets rid of foreign things in the body, like splinters, abscesses, bad odours and urates.' And, in another sentence I added: 'Elderly people, without exception, need Silica twice daily.' But it is also very important to know that Silica will eliminate foreign matter from the body that is non-functional. So beware if you have metal plates, pipes or securing screws or tubes in the body – discuss this aspect of Silica with your doctor, as this tissue salt will dissolve any metal or foreign body within the human body, even breast implants.

Ailments treated

The head

Silica is undoubtedly a wonderful treatment for anything to do with the head. After a stroke Silica is needed to absorb the haematoma. And, in more general terms, it promotes a thick growth of hair by stimulating hair follicles – even in baldness. It also treats dandruff, retards split ends and improves the condition of dull, lustreless hair. It also helps to control falling hair and generally keeps the scalp healthy. This tissue salt serves to disperse lumps and nodules on the scalp and, by the way, your nails will improve at the same time.

If there is a chronic headache that won't seem to budge, Silica is gently soothing. This type of headache can be accompanied by dizziness, nausea and it usually starts at around noon and continues until the evening with spells of forgetfulness and much irritability. Two tablets taken four to six (even 10) times throughout the day will alleviate these symptoms. Silica is also needed for a very young baby whose fontanelle is open for too long, as it will stimulate bone growth. Give the baby six drops of Silica twice a day in a teaspoon of water.

The eyes and ears

If eyes appear deeply sunken, or if there's an involuntary twitching of the eyelids, Silica will help. It will also clear red eyelids or a stye on the eyelid. And, for cataracts, and for tear ducts that are blocked, this tissue salt is a prime remedy when taken in conjunction with Calc. Fluor. Take two tablets of each three to four times a day.

The lens of the eye contains a high concentration of Silica, and when there is a disturbance, as in cataracts, Silica taken three or four times a day will help to correct the imbalance. Silica assists in the dispersion of any thick nasal catarrh discharge and, often in the ears, where it is thick and yellowish green, or, if there is deafness due to the discharge, or dullness of hearing. Take two tablets of Silica four times a day, to clear the infection. The same dose will alleviate over-sensitivity to both noise or bright light.

The mouth

For gum boils and pyorrhoea, for sores that develop on the corners of the mouth, or when mouth ulcers occur or teeth and gums feel sore, take Silica. Also, when gums are ulcerated and spongy or you have an infectious abscess, or if water tastes unpleasant and the breath smells (especially in the morning) Silica with Calc. Sulph. and Nat. Sulph. is definitely needed. Dissolve six Silica tablets in ½ a glass of warm water, swirl it around the mouth and gargle with it twice a day and, at the same time take two tablets of Silica three or four times during the day. This same dose can be used after a tooth extraction, especially if there is any doubt that a piece of tooth may have splintered and been left behind. Silica will expel it from the socket.

The skeleton

For weak or diseased bones, caries of the bones, to strengthen the spine and to ease backache – especially lumbago and sciatica, Silica is needed, two tablets four times a day. The same dose can be taken to alleviate fatigue and weariness associated with aching legs and feet, also for swelling and pain in the feet and for any swelling that persists.

Any general debilitating condition, such as hip joint disease or stiffness, and for all conditions as a result of poor nourishment or poor posture, two tablets of Silica should be taken two to four times a day. This dosage is also recommended for the pain associated with rheumatism, arthritis and for chronic synovitis. In cases of chronic weak ankles, hard tumours and the painful anchylosing spondylitis that affects the spine, and 'arthritic concretions' – literally stiffening into cement – and for osteoporosis all these ailments will be considerably relieved by taking Silica with Calc. Phos. and Nat. Mur. Take two tablets of each two to four times a day.

Digestive system

For burning indigestion and discomfort or with poor nourishment and a defective assimilation of food, two tablets of Silica taken frequently will make life more tolerable. Lack of Silica is evident by a protruding stomach on a thin child or on a thin elderly person indicating their inability to assimilate their food adequately. If there is heartburn and discomfort and diarrhoea – Silica was known as one of the greatest chronic diarrhoea remedies during the American civil war.

ℋ*aemorrhoids and anal cracks*

In cases of *constipation*, where it is difficult to expel the stool (a condition called spasm of sphincter ani) and to help heal anal fissures and fistulas which are usually accompanied by bleeding sores and cracks around the anus, take two tablets of Silica three to six times a day. The same dose will ease the pain of itchy *sore piles*. Make a *soothing lotion* especially for anal sores and piles by dissolving six tablets of Silica in ½ a cup of warm water and apply to the area frequently. Alternatively, a *cream* can be made for haemorrhoids (piles) and anal fissures using the respective tissue salts in liquid form: in ½ a cup of good quality aqueous cream, mix in 20 drops Silica, 10 drops of Calc. Fluor. and 10 drops of Ferrum Phos. Apply to the area frequently. Keep the cream in a sealed screw-top jar when not in use.

Respiratory system

Silica is needed for those slow to heal infections such as tonsillitis, pneumonia, bronchitis and asthma – all with mucous accumulation. Two tablets of Silica taken six to 10 times a day will greatly relieve these symptoms.

Infections that start in the throat and go up into the nose and then settle in the chest and clear slowly, all need Silica. Also, if this pattern of infection is reoccurring and you just can not get free of bout after bout of 'flu, Silica taken frequently with Ferrum Phos. and Kali. Mur. will clear the situation.

Note: Do not take Silica for TB as it could spread any remaining TB spores within the body during its role of waste clearing and the dispersing could start up new infections.

Female problems

Silica works effectively in clearing up a thick vaginal discharge or it disperses an abscess and hard lumps – in fact it is effective for any inflammation in the breasts, including painful nipples. It also treats premenstrual constipation and that cold, shivery feeling before a period, and it also works well to cure chronic cystitis. It even treats contagious sexually transmitted diseases like syphilis

94

and gonorrhoea. All these ailments will respond to taking two tablets of Silica, two to six times a day, depending on the severity of the ailment.

Male problems

Silica taken four to six times a day is vital to correcting such ailments as prostate problems and sexually transmitted diseases like chronic gonorrhoea, herpes infections and skin eruptions in the groin and inner thighs.

The skin

Silica improves the condition of the skin by helping to clear blind spots or pimples that don't come to a head – those bumps and lumps just under the surface, even subcutaneous cysts. It also works on open or infected skin such as acne, boils and abscesses. Take this tissue salt for skin that heals slowly, with much scarring and where there is keloid formation on wounds. It will also help when skin is fragile, flaking and peeling, or there are dry painful cracks, such as on the fingers during winter. It can reduce surface wrinkles and improve the skin's appearance when it has no lustre – hair and nails too. It also helps to quickly disperse bad bruising. In all these cases Silica is needed, take two tablets two to four times a day.

In conditions where the skin has an unpleasant odour with lots of bad smelling perspiration under arms and on the feet, Silica, when taken with Calc. Sulph. and Nat. Phos., will clear the problem. Take two tablets of each three to four times a day.

Other symptoms

- In the frenetic world we live in, stress levels reach huge proportions, and it is very important to know that Silica is an anti-stress salt.

O̸ccupational diseases

Another, and most impressive use of Silica is for treating occupational diseases experienced by those who are employed in stone works, coal mines – miners generally – where the dust gets into the lungs and lodges there and no amount of coughing can clear it. The same applies to those who work in the painting and decorating industry – painters, especially spray painters and also potters, who are likely to breath in fine particles of glaze dust. Remember that Silica is the 'surgeon', clearing waste products from the body.

- Silica is also when boils or carbuncles keep recurring or abscesses and neglected injuries fester and suppurate.
- If there is chronic neuralgia, helped by a warm poultice, or when there are copious night sweats, or too much or too little perspiration – Silica provides great relief.
- For hot flushes at night during menopause, Silica is a lifesaver.

For all the above conditions, take two tablets four to 10 times a day, depending on the severity of the problem.

Silica – the 'peacemaker'

Dr. Carey and Dr. Perry state that mental abstraction, despondence and general disgust with life arise from insufficient Silica. In their book, Dr. Carey says: 'a deficiency of Silica in the connective tissue, between the cerebrum and the cerebellum, produces a mental condition in which thinking is difficult. Warfare among nations and people, family quarrels and the attraction that any kind of fight has for the average person, is entirely due to the inharmonious state of the brain cells.' It really is quite alarming to think that there is an internal conflict going on in the blood in the brain all the time – a condition that Dr. Carey refers to as 'the war of the cerebral cells.' And, if these cells don't get the right nutrients, it is no wonder disease and lack of harmony within and without is the order of the day.

- In the treatment of alcoholism, Silica is vitally important. Or, even if you drink moderately, this tissue salt should be taken regularly because Silica can help to regulate chemical imbalances caused by the alcohol. But no amount of Silica can stop the damage if heavy drinking continues.
- The action of Silica in the digestion process is to prevent malabsorption of food. Without Silica there is consequent malnutrition and damage to the nerves in the digestive tract. Alcohol can cause chronic malabsorption, effecting the stomach lining that is often perpetually raw and bleeding. If you take a painkiller, this will only exacerbate the condition. Think about it before it is too late.
- Silica is also used to control bed-wetting, one to two tablets taken every 30 minutes before bedtime for about two hours.
- Do you have difficulty getting to sleep at night? Perhaps you experience restless symptoms of jerking limbs and twitching just before going to sleep. Silica and warmth can ease this involuntary action! Try Mag. Phos. with Silica in a little warm water – use also to treat bed-wetting in a restless child.
- Another extraordinary ability of Silica concerns the nails. Applied topically, it is able to clear fungus and ridges and white spots plus any malformation of both finger and toenails. It can also clear up fungal infections of the skin and ingrown toenails that are not caused by ill-fitting shoes. Make a *lotion* comprising six tablets of Silica, dissolved in ½ a cup of warm water, mixed with a few drops of tea tree oil. Apply frequently, and take two tablets of Silica three times a day.
- Another useful application is to take Silica before and after any type of vaccination. It helps to soothe and clear the introduced infection.
- Some doctors are using Silica to help epileptics and to build up a malnourished and retarded child. It is also being given in conjunction with Mag. Phos. to ease cramps in the calves and feet. For children and the elderly who have tremors and convulsions, Silica will steady them and become supportive.
- People who have a generally angry disposition that involves irritability and being uncooperative, obstinate, ill-humoured,

97

with often an aversion for work, and also those who tend to anger quickly and become easily agitated and over-excitable – they all need Silica.

- One miraculous thing Silica can do is to save you from that awful sinking feeling where you suddenly have to sit down as though the plug has been pulled, literally draining you of all energy. This condition is usually explained as 'a drop in your blood sugar level'. Two tablets of Silica will right that wobble and get you up and going speedily.

- If you are a 'chilly' person, quick to feel the cold and don't warm up easily, you need Silica.

- Silica comes from the seabed and from rock crystal or quartz. Silica and Calc. Fluor. are both used in the manufacture of glass lenses and both are needed in the body to healthily maintain the lenses of the eye. We need to understand how vitally important these mineral salts are!

- And finally, remember if you are over 50, Silica needs to be taken twice daily!

Secondary and complementary salts

Calc. Sulph. works well with Silica as both are cleansing salts, and Mag. Phos. with Silica also is a happy blend as Silica distributes both calcium and magnesium properly, especially when there is rapid growth and development in a young person or rapid changes in the elderly.

Herbs that contain Silica

- Dandelion: a bone and teeth builder that is rich in vitamins A, B, C and D. It is also an excellent diuretic, liver and digestive tonic and an anti-rheumatic of note. Eat at least three leaves a day, fresh from an organically grown plant in a mixed salad. Dandelion is a superb anti-ageing herb.

- Stinging nettle: a diuretic and tonic, it contains vitamins A, B and C. It also stimulates the circulation, promotes milk flow and clears uric acid from the joints, thus making it an excellent herb for people suffering from arthritis, rheumatism and gout. Make a *tea* with a ¼ cup of fresh stinging nettle leaves to one cup of boiling water. Allow to stand for five minutes then strain.

- Californian poppy: a natural painkiller, an antispasmodic and valuable herbal medicine for treating physical and psychological conditions in children, such as bed-wetting, insomnia, anxiety and mood swings. Make a *tea* as described above for stinging nettle.
- Horsetail (*Equisetum*): one of nature's most Silica-rich herbs – you can literally hear the Silica content in it if you rub the leafless stems together. It is also an anti-inflammatory, a tissue healer and bone builder. Take horsetail as a homeopathic medicine.
- Comfrey – one of nature's miracles, it is a cell proliferator, and it strengthens, builds and heals bones. It also heals wounds and is a superb expectorant. Comfrey is rich in many minerals, especially Silica. Avoid excessive internal consumption as the pyrrolizidine alkaloids it contains have been linked to liver cancer in rats. This is a restricted herb in some countries, but I name it here as I have used comfrey to heal severe bone injuries. It is known as 'knitbone' for obvious reasons, having the ability to promote the healing of bone where not even the most sophisticated bone graft can achieve results. Discuss taking *comfrey tea* with your doctor. Use a ¼ cup of fresh leave pieces to one cup of boiling water; stand for five minutes and strain. Drink one cup no more than three times a week. The results of this tea, taken in conjunction with Silica (three tablets taken three times a day), are amazing.

Foods rich in Silica

All the tall grains – wheat maize, barley, oats, buckwheat, rice – contain Silica. This tissue salt is also found in lentils, carrots, celery, chicory, soya bean, spinach, lettuce, oranges, lemons, guavas, apricots, apples, quinces and pomegranates. Starting today, make it a rule to eat at least eight different fruits and vegetables every single day! For conditions of arthritis, gout or rheumatism, rather eat rye than wheat bread, as wheat products tend to build uric acid in the joints that makes them painful and very stiff.

The constitutional tissue salt

This is the salt most needed by people born under the astrological sign of Sagittarius, and they must take it every single day. Silica is both supportive and strengthening as Sagittarians can become depleted and exhausted by mood swings, restless seeking and fiery confrontations! Silica will help them to cope and give them strength to carry on carrying on! But Silica is not only important to Sagittareans – it is essential for every single one of us. Life is becoming so stressed and so rushed, I'd go as far as saying we all need Silica every day, and twice a day when the going gets tough!

Ⱡ ilment chart

Note: Numbers next to an ailment refer to the number of the particular tissue salt(s) — see the box below. A plus (+) sign denotes combinations of tissue salts. Refer to the main text for the suggested dosage or method of application and other important information.

The 12 Tissue Salts
1. Calc. Fluor. — Calcium Fluoride (p.1)
2. Calc. Phos. — Calcium Phosphate (p.8)
3. Calc. Sulph. — Calcium Sulphate (p.16)
4. Ferrum Phos. — Ferrum Phosphoricum (p.24)
5. Kali. Mur. — Kalium Muriaticum (p.32)
6. Kali. Phos. — Kalium Phosphate (p.40)
7. Kali. Sulph. — Kalium Sulphate (p.50)
8. Mag. Phos. — Magnesium Phosphate (p.57)
9. Nat. Mur. — Natrium Muriaticum (p.65)
10. Nat. Phos. — Phosphoricum (p.75)
11. Nat. Sulph. — Natrium Sulphate (p.83)
12. Silica — Silicon Dioxide (p.91)

A
abdominal bloating 11
abrupt behaviour 11
abscess 3, 12
absent-mindedness 12
ache reliever 5
aches and pains 4
aching limbs 3

acid neutraliser 10
acid urine 10
acid/alkaline balancer 10
acidity 2 + 8 + 10
acne 2, 3, 5, 12
adenoids, swollen 2, 5
aged
  Alzheimer's disease 6, 12
  bad moods 2, 6, 9

bed sores 4, 6
blurred vision 6
cold feet 3
depression 2, 6
fear of becoming ill 2, 6
fear of dying 6
grief and adjustment to loss 2, 6
inability to concentrate 6, 9, 12
incontinence, 2, 4, 6, 8, 10
insomnia 6
irritability 6
loss of vitality and energy 6
muscle pain 6, 8
night terrors 2, 6
paralysis 6
poor memory 2, 6, 12
remorse 6
senility 6
sensation of numbness 6
suspicion of other people 2, 6, 9
tearfulness 2, 6
throbbing varicosities 3, 8
tremors and convulsions 12
ulcerated varicosities 3
weak feeling in the extremities 6, 12
weak muscle action 6, 12
withdrawing from people 2, 6
ageing 1, 6, 9, 12
aggressiveness 2, 9
ailments associated with cold, damp
  weather 1, 11
alcoholism 5, 8
allergic rhinitis 9
allergy rash 9 + 3
allergy swellings 9, 7
alopecia *see* hair loss
anaemia 2 + 4, 4, 4 + 9
anal fissures and fistulas 12 + 1 + 4

anal itch 7
anal sores 4, 12
analgesic 6 + 8
anchylosing spondylitis 12 + 2 + 9
anger 2, 6, 12
angina pectoris 6 + 8
animals, ageing 2, 12
animals, infection 4
anorexia 6, 9
antacid 10
anti-inflammatory 4 + 5
antiseptic 6
antispasmodic 2, 8
anxiety 6, 8, 11, 12
  with a fluttering heart 2, 6, 9
appetite
  hunger pangs 8
  lack of 3, 12
  ravenous 2, 3
arthritis 5, 8, 9, 12
  acute 4, 10
  chronic 4, 10
asthma 1, 5, 8 + 5, 9, 11, 12
  chronic 6 + 8, 7, 11
  nervous 6, 11, 12
astigmatism 4, 6
athlete's foot 11 + 7
autism 6, 11
aversion for work 9, 12
awkwardness 9

B

babies
  closing of fontanelle 2, 12
  colic 2, 8
  constipation 4
  cradle cap 5
  delayed dentition 1, 2
  flatulence 8

1. Calc. Fluor. (p.1)	2. Calc. Phos. (p.8)	3. Calc. Sulph. (p.16)	4. Ferrum Phos. (p.24)
5.Kali. Mur. (p.32)	6. Kali. Phos. (p.40)	7. Kali. Sulph. (p.50)	8. Mag. Phos. (p.57)
9. Nat. Mur. (p.65)	10. Nat. Phos. (p.75)	11. Nat. Sulph. (p.83)	12. Silica (p.91)

fretfulness 2
inflamed crusty vaccinations 5
inflamed gums and ulcers 5
mouth red and swollen 5 + 4
teething 4 + 2 + 8
teething with excessive salivation 9
back pain, lower 8
back strain 1 + 9
back strengthener 1
backache 2, 4, 5, 11, 12
  chronic 10
  during menstruation 7
bad breath 2, 10, 11, 11 + 2 + 12, 12
  + 3 + 11
bad temper 6
baldness 7, 9, 12
bed-wetting 4, 6
bee sting 4, 7
belching of sour gases 5, 10, 11
Bell's palsy 6
bilious fever 11
biliousness 10, 11
bitter taste in the mouth 11, 12
bladder ailments 1, 2 + 10, 3, 4, 6,
  8, 10
bloating 2, 9, 10
blocked nose 3, 7, 11
blood alkaliser 8, 10
blood and lymph cleanser 5
blood cleanser 3, 10
blood poisoning 7, 10, 12
blood sugar, high 10, 11
blood sugar, low 4, 11, 12
blood vessels, to strengthen 4, 8
body odour 10, 12 + 3 + 10, 6 +
  10 + 12
boils 3, 5, 12
bones, weak or diseased 2, 12

bowel cramps 8
bowel, burning pain in lower part 7
brain tonic 6, 9, 12
brain-fatigue 6, 12
breastfeeding 6, 9
breasts, abscesses and hard lumps 12
breathlessness 8, 11
bronchitis 2, 7, 12, 2 + 5, 4 + 3 + 7
  with much production of phlegm 5
  with thick yellow sputum 3
bruising 12
bumps under the skin 1
bunions 1, 2
burnout 6 + 8
burns, minor 3, 4, 5
bursitis 5
butterflies in the stomach 2, 6

C

calming 2, 6, 12
cancer 3, 6, 7
  intestinal 6, 7 + 4
  of the face 7 + 4
  of the nose 7 + 4
  uterine 7 + 4
  vaginal 6, 7 + 4
cancer formula 5 + 6 + 7 + 4
cancer protector 7 + 3
candida 5
carbuncle 3, 12
caries of the bones 1, 12
cataracts 1 + 2, 9, 12 + 2
catarrh 3, 5 + 4
  mucous 5
  thick green 11
cell builder 2, 7, 12
cell cleanser 11, 12
cellulite 9, 11
chest infections 4, 7, 12

1. Calc. Fluor. (p.1)	2. Calc. Phos. (p.8)	3. Calc. Sulph. (p.16)	4. Ferrum Phos. (p.24)
5.Kali. Mur. (p.32)	6. Kali. Phos. (p.40)	7. Kali. Sulph. (p.50)	8. Mag. Phos. (p.57)
9. Nat. Mur. (p.65)	10. Nat. Phos. (p.75)	11. Nat. Sulph. (p.83)	12. Silica (p.91)

chest pains 6 + 8, 8
chest tightness 1
chilblains 2
children
  asthma 4, 6 + 8
  aiding mental development 2
  aiding physical development 2
  bad temper 2
  bed-wetting 2, 8, 12 + 8
  chicken pox 5, 7
  congestion in ears, nose and
    throat 7
  diarrhoea 3
  eczema 7, 10
  erratic behaviour 1, 12
  food allergies 4
  fretfulness 2 + 8
  growing children 1, 2
  growing pains 2, 4, 2 + 6 + 8
  headache 2
  hyperactive 6, 10
  infection 4
  infection due to vaccination 12
  instability 1, 12
  itchy chicken pox blisters 9
  lack of concentration 1, 2, 6
  measles 5, 7
  mumps 5
  nightmares 2, 6
  poor appetite 2
  poor concentration 2
  poor diet 10
  poor memory 2
  projectile vomiting 4
  rashes 7
  residual cough 7
  restless sleep 2, 4, 6, 8, 10
  rough, hoarse voice 2

scarlet fever 5
slow mental development 2
sore ears 4
sore joints 2 + 6 + 8
sour belching 4, 10
tremors and convulsions 1, 12
twitching limbs 2, 12
vomiting undigested milk 4, 10
chilliness 2 + 4
chronic aches 5, 10, 12
circulation 1, 2 + 4, 6 + 4
cirrhosis of the liver 5
cold extremities 2, 9
cold sweats 8
colds 1, 2, 4 + 3 + 7, 5, 5 + 4, 7, 9
colic 7, 8, 9, 10, 11
colon, inflammation 6
complexion, pasty 2
concussion 4, 11
conditions resulting from poor
  diet 9, 12
conditions resulting from poor
  posture 3, 12
confusion 6
congestion 4
  nose, throat and chest 4 + 7
  in pelvic area 5
  lymphatic 5
constipation 1, 3, 9, 11, 12
  premenstrual 12
convalescence 2 + 4, 5
convulsions 4, 8, 11
coping, unable 2, 4, 6
corns 1, 12
cough
  chronic 2, 4, 6 + 8, 7
  dry 5, 8
  irritating 1, 5

1. Calc. Fluor. (p.1)	2. Calc. Phos. (p.8)	3. Calc. Sulph. (p.16)	4. Ferrum Phos. (p.24)
5.Kali. Mur. (p.32)	6. Kali. Phos. (p.40)	7. Kali. Sulph. (p.50)	8. Mag. Phos. (p.57)
9. Nat. Mur. (p.65)	10. Nat. Phos. (p.75)	11. Nat. Sulph. (p.83)	12. Silica (p.91)

productive 1, 3 + 7
spasmodic 1, 8
tight 6, 11
with thick phlegm and yellow
sputum 11
cracks around the anus 9
cramps
associated with muscle control 8
associated with playing a musical
instrument 8
in calves and feet 12 + 8
severe 6, 8, 12
cravings
cold sweet drinks 11
for food, even after a large meal 6
salty and savoury foods 2 + 9, 3
sugar 7 + 8
sweet cold drinks 8
croup 4 + 7, 5, 8 + 5
cuts 3, 4
cystic fibrosis 5 + 4
cystitis 4 + 10, 5 + 4, 7, 10, 12
with yellow discharge 7, 11, 12
cysts 1, 12

D

dandruff 3, 5, 7, 10, 12
debility 9, 12
decongestant 5, 11
demotivation 1, 12
depression 4, 6, 9, 11
as a result of bad weather 1, 6, 9
clinical 9, 11
manic 2, 6, 9, 11
postnatal 9
dermatitis 7, 9
despair 6, 9, 11
desperation 4
despondence 4, 11, 12

detoxify 3
diabetes 9, 11
late-onset 8
diarrhoea 3, 4, 8, 10, 12
bad smelling 6
sour-smelling 10
thin, watery, painless 9, 11
watery 9, 11
yellow 7, 11
digestion of fats 6
digestive problems
allergies 5
belching, sour 11
indigestion 1, 2, 6, 9, 10
indigestion, burning 2 + 8 + 10,
3, 12
indigestion, nervous 6
painful sour reflux 10
spasms 2 + 8
stomach cramps 8
stomach lining, raw and bleeding 12
stomach ulcers 3, 10
stomach, feeling of heat or
churning 10
see also Diarrhoea; Stools
digestive tonic 10 + 11
disability, after a fall or concussion 8
disability, chronic 8
disappointment 6
dislike of otherwise favourite
foods 10
distraction 9
disturbing dreams 1
dizziness 4, 6 + 8, 10, 11
dread of noise 6
dreams, bad 6, 12
dribbling 9
dropsy 5

1. Calc. Fluor. (p.1)	2. Calc. Phos. (p.8)	3. Calc. Sulph. (p.16)	4. Ferrum Phos. (p.24)
5.Kali. Mur. (p.32)	6. Kali. Phos. (p.40)	7. Kali. Sulph. (p.50)	8. Mag. Phos. (p.57)
9. Nat. Mur. (p.65)	10. Nat. Phos. (p.75)	11. Nat. Sulph. (p.83)	12. Silica (p.91)

drug addiction 6, 9, 10
dry mouth 1, 12
dull, lustreless hair 12
dyslexia 2, 6
dyspepsia 6, 10

E

Ears
blocked 2, 3, 7
buzzing sounds 2, 6, 9
deafness accompanied by anxiety
and extreme nervous tension 8, 9,
10, 12
deafness due to chronic catarrh
7, 11
deafness due to discharge 11, 12
deafness due to swelling 4, 7
earache 2, 3, 4, 11
earache with thick, yellow discharge
or dark wax 7
earache, with sharp, shooting pains
4, 8
hot, stuffy, itchy 9
infection, recurring 4, 5
inflamed 4
noises 2, 9
over-sensitivity to noise 12
pulsating or twitching 6
ringing 2, 3, 8, 9
swollen 6, 11
thick, yellowish-green discharge
11, 12
tinnitis 1, 3
wax production 3
eczema 3, 6, 7, 10, 11
chronic 5, 9 + 3
dry and scaly 5, 9
facial 9 + 3
itching and weeping 9

vesicular 5
weeping 1, 5
elderly, rapid changes 3, 8, 12
eliminator 3
emotional distress 6
emotional tension 6
emphysema 1, 5
endocrine imbalance 9
energy, lack of 2
enlarged finger joints 1
enuresis 4 + 6
epilepsy 4, 6, 12
exam-time worries, tension and fear
2, 6, 10
excessive dryness 9
excessive moisture 9
excessive salivation 6, 9
excessive thirst, or craving for salty
foods 9
exhaustion 6 + 8
eyes
abnormal dilation or constriction of
pupils 8
aching 2, 6
blocked tear ducts 12 + 2
bloodshot 4
blurred vision 1, 3, 6, 8
burning sensation 4
conjunctivitis 1 + 2 + 9, 2, 3, 4, 10
crusts forming at corners 5, 7, 10
deeply sunken 12
delayed focusing 1
double vision with a headache 9
dry scratchy and painful 9
dry sensation 6
eyelids, itchy 7, 9
eyelids, red 7, 10, 12
eyelid, stye 12

---

1. Calc. Fluor. (p.1)	2. Calc. Phos. (p.8)	3. Calc. Sulph. (p.16)	4. Ferrum Phos. (p.24)
5.Kali. Mur. (p.32)	6. Kali. Phos. (p.40)	7. Kali. Sulph. (p.50)	8. Mag. Phos. (p.57)
9. Nat. Mur. (p.65)	10. Nat. Phos. (p.75)	11. Nat. Sulph. (p.83)	12. Silica (p.91)

eyelids, swollen 7
eyelids, twitching 8
failing vision 7
fatigue from computer screen 6
feeling of pressure 1
flashes of colour 6
flashing lights 2
flickering 10
floating black spots 6
fluttering tic 8
glaucoma 6, 9
granulation on eyelids 5
gritty 4
'halo' effects 6
infection 3
inflamed 4
inflammation of conjunctiva 7
involuntary twitching 12
itchy, dry 9
nervous tick 1
over-sensitivity to bright light 2, 8, 12
pains 1, 6
pink eyes *see* conjunctivitis
poor focus 11
puffiness 9
red, bloodshot 6
retinal discharge 5
spots on cornea 1 + 2
squinting 8
strained 1
tears, continual 3
thick yellow discharge 11
twitches 2
ulcers 1 + 2, 2, 3
visual distortion 2, 7
watery 3, 9
weakening 6

exam-time worries 2, 4, 6, 8, 10
exhaustion 2, 9, 10

F

fainting 2, 4, 10
faintness 2, 6 + 8
fatigue 1, 2, 9, 10, 12
fatty deposits, to disperse 2
fear or dread 6, 11, 12
feel-good-all-over remedy 2 + 4 + 6
feeling of fullness 7
feeling of suffocation 7
feet
  bunions 1, 2
  burning 3
  burning soles 11
  chilled 2, 4, 9, 11, 12
  corns 1, 12
  cramps 2, 8, 9
  heel ache 2, 8
  ingrown toenails 12
  itchy 7, 8
  numbness 2
  smelly 6, 12
  swollen 11, 12
fever 4, 9
fever blisters 3, 9
fibroids 2, 9
fibrositis 10
flatulence 2, 5, 6, 8
  after consuming cold drinks 8, 11
  sulphur-smelling 7, 8
flexibility, to promote 1, 12
florid complexion 4
'flu 4, 7
  chronic 12 + 4 + 5
'flu formula 1 + 4 + 5 + 9 + 11
flushed face 4

---

1. Calc. Fluor. (p.1)	2. Calc. Phos. (p.8)	3. Calc. Sulph. (p.16)	4. Ferrum Phos. (p.24)
5. Kali. Mur. (p.32)	6. Kali. Phos. (p.40)	7. Kali. Sulph. (p.50)	8. Mag. Phos. (p.57)
9. Nat. Mur. (p.65)	10. Nat. Phos. (p.75)	11. Nat. Sulph. (p.83)	12. Silica (p.91)

flushes, hot 4, 9, 10
food allergies 4
food intolerance 4
food cravings 3, 10
forgetfulness 4, 8
fractures 1 + 2
frequent urge to urinate 8
fungal infections 6, 12
fungoid inflammation of the joints 7

G
gall bladder problems 4, 10, 11
gallstones 10, 11
gangrene 6, 4
gassy bowel 6, 10
gastric fever 5, 10
gastric tract, acute infection 4, 6
gastritis 6
gastro-enteritis 6, 9
genital herpes 3
genital itch 11
getting rid of emotional 'waste' 5
glandular fever 5
glandular tonic 5
gloominess 2, 6, 9
gonorrhoea 9, 12
gout 1, 10 + 11 + 4
green stick fractures 2
grief 6, 9
growth supporter 2
growths 1, 4, 12
Guillain-Barré syndrome *see* yuppie
  flu
gums
  bleeding 2 + 1, 3, 6
  boils 3, 4, 7, 12
  infectious abscess 6, 9, 12
  inflamed 2 + 1, 4
  painful 12

raised pale patches 5, 6
spongy 5, 6
ulcerated and spongy 12
ulcers 4, 9

H
haemophilia 4, 11
haemorrhoids 1, 4, 5, 7, 9, 12 +
  1 + 4
hair
  falling 3, 7, 12
  lifeless, dull 3, 7
  loss 2, 3, 6, 7, 9, 12
  pulling out or tugging and
  twisting 6
  split ends 3, 12
  straggly 7, 9, 12
halitosis 6, 10, 12
hands
  chilled 2, 4, 9, 11
  clammy 2
  cramps 2
  feeling of pins and needles 2
  itchy dry skin 7, 10
  numbness 2
  stiff 5
  thick, achy finger joints 1, 9
  uncontrollable shaking 8
hard tumours 12 + 2 + 9
hatefulness 9
hay fever 6, 9
  chronic 5 + 9
head injury 11
headache 9
  accompanied by dizziness,
  nausea 12
  accompanied by sour belching and
  heartburn 10 + 11
  at back of head 6

1. Calc. Fluor. (p.1)	2. Calc. Phos. (p.8)	3. Calc. Sulph. (p.16)	4. Ferrum Phos. (p.24)
5.Kali. Mur. (p.32)	6. Kali. Phos. (p.40)	7. Kali. Sulph. (p.50)	8. Mag. Phos. (p.57)
9. Nat. Mur. (p.65)	10. Nat. Phos. (p.75)	11. Nat. Sulph. (p.83)	12. Silica (p.91)

caused by being overheated 9
caused by hot, stuffy room 7
caused by muscular tension 8
caused by nervous tension 8
chronic 12
congestive 4
from loss of sleep 6 + 8
from too much work 6 + 8
nauseous 11 + 10
neuralgic 8
sinus 7
throbbing 4
with blocked sinuses 5
with coldness 2
with confusion 6
with decreased libido 9
with dizziness 6
with sharp, shooting pains 8
with spells of forgetfulness and
    irritability 12
with stabbing pain over one eye 8
heart beat, irregular 6, 8, 9
heartburn 5, 8, 9, 10, 11, 12
heart palpitations 2, 4, 6, 8
heart tonic 6 + 8
heaviness of limb 5
heel ache 2, 8
hepatitis 3, 5, 11
herpes 3, 4, 9, 12
herpes blisters 7
hiatus hernia 1
hiccups 1, 8, 8 + 5, 11
high blood pressure 4 + 6
high temperature 4
hip pain 8, 11
hip joint disease 12
hives 9, 10
hopelessness 2, 6, 9, 11

hot flushes 4, 9
hyperactivity 6, 8
hypersensitivity 6, 9
hysterical spasms 2, 9

I

ill-humour 12
immune dysfunction 5 + 4, 6, 9
impatience 9
impotence 4, 6, 9
inability to get started in the
    mornings 11
incontinence 4, 11
    when sneezing or coughing 10 + 2
    + 6 + 9
indecisiveness 1, 6
indifference 9
indigestion 1, 2, 6, 9, 10
    burning 2 + 8 + 10, 3, 12
    nervous 6
infection 4, 5
infertility 3, 9
inflammation (first stage) 4
inflammation (second stage) 5
inflammation (third stage) 7
influenza 4, 5, 9, 11
injuries, where septic conditions
    develop 6
insect bites 3, 8, 9, 10
insomnia 3 + 2 + 6, 4, 6, 8, 9, 10, 11
intolerance of tight clothing around
    abdomen 11
irritability 4, 6, 9, 11, 12
irritable bowel syndrome 1, 2 + 6 +
    11, 8
itchy anus 10
itchy shins 10

1. Calc. Fluor. (p.1)	2. Calc. Phos. (p.8)	3. Calc. Sulph. (p.16)	4. Ferrum Phos. (p.24)
5.Kali. Mur. (p.32)	6. Kali. Phos. (p.40)	7. Kali. Sulph. (p.50)	8. Mag. Phos. (p.57)
9. Nat. Mur. (p.65)	10. Nat. Phos. (p.75)	11. Nat. Sulph. (p.83)	12. Silica (p.91)

J

jangled nerves 6, 9, 12
jarring falls 11
jaundice 3, 5, 10, 11
joints
  aching 3, 4 + 10, 5, 7, 11
  cracking 9, 10, 11
  painful 3, 7, 10, 11
joylessness 2, 6, 9

K

kidney pain 3, 10
kidney stones 2 + 10, 11
kidney weakness 10

L

leucorrhea 3, 5, 9 + 2
leukaemia 11
libido, poor 2, 4, 9
limb jerking 8
liver
  cleanser 3, 10, 11
  disease, chronic 8
  distended and tender to the
    touch 11
  problems 10, 11
  sluggish 5
liver spots 11
liverishness 3, 10, 11 + 10
low blood pressure 2 + 9, 11 + 4
low spirits 2, 6, 9
lower back pain 1, 12
lumbago 2, 12
lungs, inflamed 4, 6 + 8
lymph glands, swollen 2, 5

M

malabsorption of food 12
malaria 11

measles 4, 5
melancholia 2, 6, 11
memory loss 2, 3, 6
menopause
  florid complexion 4
  hot flushes 4, 7, 8, 12
  night sweats 4
  regulator 2
  sudden increase in blood pressure
    4 + 6
  swollen feet or hands 4
  vertigo 4
menstruation
  cramps 2 + 8, 4 + 8, 5 + 8, 6, 8
  flow, excessive 1, 4, 5 + 4, 9
  flow, too thick 1
  flow, with bearing down pains 1
  flow, with large, dark clots 1, 5
  heavy bloated feeling in the lower
    abdomen 9
  regulator 2
  mood swings 6, 8, 9
  irregular 2, 4, 9
  suppressed 2, 7
mental abstraction 12
mental confusion 8
mental exertion 10
mental fatigue 2, 3, 6
mental fuzziness 7, 10, 11
mental weakness due to head injury
  and concussion 11
metabolism 6
middle-ear infection 1, 5 + 4
migraine 8, 11
moodiness 2, 8
mood-lifter formula 11 + 6 + 2
morning sickness 4, 5, 10, 11
mosquito bites 8

1. Calc. Fluor. (p.1)	2. Calc. Phos. (p.8)	3. Calc. Sulph. (p.16)	4. Ferrum Phos. (p.24)
5.Kali. Mur. (p.32)	6. Kali. Phos. (p.40)	7. Kali. Sulph. (p.50)	8. Mag. Phos. (p.57)
9. Nat. Mur. (p.65)	10. Nat. Phos. (p.75)	11. Nat. Sulph. (p.83)	12. Silica (p.91)

mouth
  bad taste 2
  bitter taste 6
  burning sensation 11
  cracks at corners 9
  dry 3, 5, 9
  inflamed, swollen area 4
  sores that develop in corners 12
  thrush 5
  ulcers 3, 12
mucous, productive 3, 4
mucous membranes, discharge 7
muddled thinking 7
mumps 5, 9
muscle twitching 8
muscular aches and pains 3, 4, 8
muscular tension 8 + 2

N
nail builder 2, 12
nails
  flaking and peeling 7
  fungal infection 7, 9, 12
  ridges and white spots 12
  thickening and distorted growth
    7, 12
nappy rash 3
nasal catarrh 2, 5, 9, 12
nasal discharge 3 + 7
  itchy, cream-coloured 5, 9, 10
nasal infections, chronic 4
nasal polpi 2
natural tranquilliser 1, 2 + 9, 6, 11
nausea 4, 8, 9, 10
  from over-indulgence 5 + 11
  violent 8
nephritis 10
nerve and muscle relaxant 8
nerves

degeneration 6
nutrient 6
tonic 6
nervous breakdown 6
nervous exhaustion 8 + 6
nervous system, stabilise 2, 6
nervous tension 6, 8
neuralgia
  around eyes 8
  chronic 12
  of face and jaw 7 + 8
  pains 6
night sweats 12
night terrors 6, 8, 10
nightmares 1, 6, 8, 11
nipples, painful 12
nose bleeds 4, 9
nose, blocked 7
nose, clear streaming 4
nose, dry 9
nose, obstructed swollen 6
numbness in extremities 4, 6
nymphomania 9 + 2

O
obesity 2, 9, *see also* slimming
occupational diseases 12
osteoporosis 2, 12 + 2 + 9
otitis media 8
over-anxiety 6
over-excitement 6, 9
overheating 4
over-indulgence in alcohol 9
over-stimulation 6
overwork 6
oxygenator 4, 4 + 7

P
pacing to and fro 8

1. Calc. Fluor. (p.1)	2. Calc. Phos. (p.8)	3. Calc. Sulph. (p.16)	4. Ferrum Phos. (p.24)
5.Kali. Mur. (p.32)	6. Kali. Phos. (p.40)	7. Kali. Sulph. (p.50)	8. Mag. Phos. (p.57)
9. Nat. Mur. (p.65)	10. Nat. Phos. (p.75)	11. Nat. Sulph. (p.83)	12. Silica (p.91)

pain 8 + 2, 12
  associated with ovulation 8
  premenstrual 8
  rheumatic 7
  sharp, shooting or constricting
    6, 8
  shifting or wandering 6, 7
painkiller 8
palpitations 4
panic attacks 4, 6, 7 + 4
paralysis 6
Parkinson's disease 4, 6, 8
personality changes 6, 8, 9
perspiration, too much or too little
  3, 12
phlegm, with albuminous nose
  mucous 2
pigmentation 3, 5
piles *see* haemorrhoids
pimples 2, 3, 7
  that don't come to a head 12
  watery 9 + 3
pink eyes *see* Eyes: conjunctivitis
pleurisy 5
PMT (premenstrual tension) 6 + 8
pneumonia 2 + 5, 3, 5, 7, 12
poor circulation 4
poor concentration 2, 8, 11
poor memory 12
positive attitude 2
post-nasal drip 1, 2, 9
posture, bad 2, 12
pregnancy
  baby refusing the breast 9
  cracked, sore nipples 9
  cramp 2
  discomfort 2
  false labour pains 8
  haemorrhoids 9

hair loss 9
headache 2
incontinence 4 + 10 + 11, 9 + 4
morning sickness 4, 9, 10
nausea 4
over-production of milk 11
pain during childbirth 8
protracted labour 6
shaky, 'gone' feeling in the
  stomach 9
slow labour 9
temporary abhorrence of certain
  foods with nausea and vomiting 9
to carry a baby to full term 2
to develop healthy bones in babies
  2 + 8
to subdue vomiting 11
vomiting of frothy phlegm 9
promoting feelings of well-being
  2 + 6
prostate
  enlargement 1, 3
  problems 1, 5, 8, 12
prostatitis 4, 9
psoriasis 5, 7, 9
public speaking 8
pulse, rapid 4
pyorrhoea 12

Q
queasy stomach 11
quickness to anger 9

R
rashes 3, 5, 6, 7, 9, 11
rectal fissures 1 + 7
recuperation 2
reduced sexual potency 6
rejuvenator 3

1. Calc. Fluor. (p.1)	2. Calc. Phos. (p.8)	3. Calc. Sulph. (p.16)	4. Ferrum Phos. (p.24)
5. Kali. Mur. (p.32)	6. Kali. Phos. (p.40)	7. Kali. Sulph. (p.50)	8. Mag. Phos. (p.57)
9. Nat. Mur. (p.65)	10. Nat. Phos. (p.75)	11. Nat. Sulph. (p.83)	12. Silica (p.91)

respiratory ailments 3, 7, 12
respiratory tract, to strengthen 3 +
6, 7 + 4
rescue remedy 2, 4, 6
restoration 2
rheumatic pains 4, 9, 11
rheumatism 1, 2, 5, 8, 9, 11, 12
in wet cold weather 4
rickets 2, 12
rose rash 4, 10
rush of blood to the head 4

S

sadness 1, 2, 6
scabies 11
scalp
crusts 5
discharging crusts 3
dry, scaly 10
eczema 9 + 3
excessively dry 9
flakiness 2, 7
itchy 9
itchy blisters 5
lumps and nodules 12
ringworm 7
scaly crusts 9
skin eruptions 9
scar tissue 1, 2, 12
sciatica 6, 8, 10, 11, 12
scratches 3
sense of smell
loss of (in absence of catarrh)
8 + 6
loss of 7 + 9 + 11
sense of taste, loss of 7 + 9 + 11
sensitivity to cold 9
sepsis 3, 12

sexual excesses and vices 10
sexual problems 8
shaking 8, 12
shin soreness 2
shingles 6 + 8, 9 + 8
special formula 9 + 5 + 6 + 2 + 4
shivering 8
short temper 11
shortness of breath on exertion 4
shoulder pains 5
shoulders, stiff, aching 7
side-effects of aspirin and other
painkillers 3 + 8
sinuses
aching 2
blocked 3, 7
sinusitis 5, 9
allergic 4, 9
skin
age spots 7
all-over itch 8, 10
blisters and watery discharge 9
burning feeling 9 + 3
chapped 1
cracked 1, 12
eruptions 3, 12
fissures around nails 1
fragile, flaking and peeling 12
freckles 7, 11
fungal infections 7, 12
growths 1
itchy 7, 11
liver spots 7
lubricator 7
oily patches on face 9
peeling 5
persistent discharge 3
reducing surface wrinkles 12

---

1. Calc. Fluor. (p.1)	2. Calc. Phos. (p.8)	3. Calc. Sulph. (p.16)	4. Ferrum Phos. (p.24)
5.Kali. Mur. (p.32)	6. Kali. Phos. (p.40)	7. Kali. Sulph. (p.50)	8. Mag. Phos. (p.57)
9. Nat. Mur. (p.65)	10. Nat. Phos. (p.75)	11. Nat. Sulph. (p.83)	12. Silica (p.91)

rejuvenator 10 + 2 + 7
rough, red skin 2, 7
scaly eruptions on moist skin 7
scarring with keloid formation 12
shaving rash 3, 7
suppuration 3
that heals slowly 12
thin, white, scaly patches 9
watery secretions 11
yellowing 10, 11
sleep
  anxious with aching shoulders and
    neck 2 + 4 + 6 + 8 + 10
  grinding teeth 10
  insomnia 3 + 2 + 6, 4, 6, 8, 9,
    10, 11
  restless 3, 4, 6, 8, 10
  restless with anxiety-ridden
    dreams 11
  restless with chilled feet 3 + 2
    + 6
  restless with much twitching and
    jerking 2, 4, 6, 8, 9, 10, 12 + 8
  snoring 5, 11
sleeping sickness 9
sleeplessness *see* insomnia
slimming 1 + 2
slow and difficult thought
  patterns 12
small pox 7
smoking, to stop 10 + 11
sneezing constantly 9
snoring 5, 11
social withdrawal 2, 6, 12
sorrow 2, 6
spasm 8 + 2
  bronchial 8
  of mucous membrane 8
  of sphincter ani 12

spasmodic cramps 8
spastic colon 8
spastic-type rigors 8
spine, strengthening 12
sprains 4
squinting. 8
stammering 8
stiff neck 8 + 6
stiff shoulders 4
stiffness 4, 5, 10, 11, 12
  due to coldness 2
  due to poor circulation 2
stings from wasps, bees or scorpions
  8, 9, 10
stomach
  cramps 8
  feeling of heat or churning 10
  lining, raw and bleeding 12
  ulcers 3, 10
stools
  burning 10
  difficulty to expel 12
  dry and straw-coloured 3
  thin, black 7
  undigested 4
  with signs of blood 4
strains 4
stress 6, 8 + 6, 9, 12
stroke 4, 6, 8
to absorb the haematoma 12
stuffiness in nose, throat and chest
  5, 7
stumbling 6
stuttering 6, 8
'St. Vitus dance' 8
suicidal tendencies 6, 11
sunstroke 4, 8, 9
suppuration reducer 3
sweating 9

1. Calc. Fluor. (p.1)	2. Calc. Phos. (p.8)	3. Calc. Sulph. (p.16)	4. Ferrum Phos. (p.24)
5.Kali. Mur. (p.32)	6. Kali. Phos. (p.40)	7. Kali. Sulph. (p.50)	8. Mag. Phos. (p.57)
9. Nat. Mur. (p.65)	10. Nat. Phos. (p.75)	11. Nat. Sulph. (p.83)	12. Silica (p.91)

sweating caused by fearfulness 8
swelling 12
  ankles 9
  hands 4
  feet 4
  limbs 9
synovitis, chronic 4, 8, 12
syphilis 9, 12

T
tearfulness 9
  continual 3
teeth
  chattering 6
  deficient enamel 1, 4
  delayed dentition 1
  dental caries 1, 2
  difficult teething 1, 2
  impacted 2
  loose 1
  painful 12
  poorly developed
  sensitive 1
  tooth decay 1, 2 + 1
  tooth extraction, rinse 4 + 8, 12
  toothache 1, 4 + 8, 6, 8
temperature, raised 4, 9
temper tantrums 6, 8, 9, 12
tension 2, 6,
  related to sexual problems 2, 6, 8
tetanus 8
the Pill, side-effects 2
thirst 9
  insatiable 9
throat
  constricted 2, 7, 8
  inflamed or ulcerated 10
  sore 2, 3 + 7, 4 + 3 + 7, 8, 9
thrush 5, 10

tinnitis 1, 3
tiredness 4
tissue overproduction 1
tongue
  coated 3
  cracked 1
  mapped 9
  numb 2
  raised pale patches 5
  ulcers 4
  with grey-brown coating 11
  with yellowish coating 7, 10
tonic 2
toning 1, 6 + 2
tonsillitis 2, 3 + 7, 4 + 3 + 7, 12
tonsils, swollen 2, 5
Tourette's syndrome. 8
toxaemia 3
toxin eliminator 3, 10, 11, 12
tranquilliser 11 + 6 + 2 + 9
tremors 8, 12
travel sickness 6, 11
typhoid 7
typhus 7

U
ulcers, slow-healing 3
unhappiness 2, 6, 9
uplifting 6
urethra, hardening of tissue 1
urinary system
  alkaliser 10
  frequent urination 9
  frequent urination during
    pregnancy 4, 10, 11
  painful urination 8
  thin watery, colourless urine 9
  urine incontinence 4, 10, 11
  urine retention 8, 11

1. Calc. Fluor. (p.1)	2. Calc. Phos. (p.8)	3. Calc. Sulph. (p.16)	4. Ferrum Phos. (p.24)
5.Kali. Mur. (p.32)	6. Kali. Phos. (p.40)	7. Kali. Sulph. (p.50)	8. Mag. Phos. (p.57)
9. Nat. Mur. (p.65)	10. Nat. Phos. (p.75)	11. Nat. Sulph. (p.83)	12. Silica (p.91)

urine spurt, 4, 10 ,11
uterine cramps 9 + 8
uterus
  fibroids 1
  prolapsed 4
  to restore muscle tone 1

V

vaginal problems
  acid discharge10
  discharge that creates irritation 10
  discharge with burning itch 9 + 2
  discharge with loss of pubic hair
    9 + 2
  discharge with unpleasant sour
    smell 10
  sour smelling discharge 11
  thick discharge 12
  thick, white discharge 5
  vaginal dryness 9
varicose ulcers 3, 4
varicose veins 1, 4
vertigo 6 + 8, 9, 10
vindictiveness 9
voice strain or loss 4, 9
vomiting 8, 10, 11

green bitter bile 11
of sour foods ₁0
of undigested food 1

W

warts 1, 5, 7, 9, 11
waste eliminator 5
water retention 4
weak ankles, chronic 12 + 2 + 9
weakness in the legs 10
weariness 1, 5
weariness associated with aching legs
  and feet 12
weepiness 6, 8
weight gain 2
weight loss 2
whitlows 3, 11, 12
whooping cough 5, 7
worms 10, 11
worry 6
wound, slow-healing 3, 6
writer's cramp 5, 8

Y

yawning 8
yuppie 'flu 6

1. Calc. Fluor. (p.1)	2. Calc. Phos. (p.8)	3. Calc. Sulph. (p.16)	4. Ferrum Phos. (p.24)
5.Kali. Mur. (p.32)	6. Kali. Phos. (p.40)	7. Kali. Sulph. (p.50)	8. Mag. Phos. (p.57)
9. Nat. Mur. (p.65)	10. Nat. Phos. (p.75)	11. Nat. Sulph. (p.83)	12. Silica (p.91)